MAD

WITH

FREEDOM

The Political Economy of Blackness, Insanity, and
Civil Rights in the U.S. South, 1840–1940

ÉLODIE EDWARDS-GROSSI

LOUISIANA STATE UNIVERSITY PRESS
BATON ROUGE

Published by Louisiana State University Press
lsupress.org

DESIGNER: Michelle A. Neustrom
TYPEFACE: Arno Pro

An earlier version of chapter 2 first appeared as "Truth in Numbers?
Emancipation, Race, and Federal Census Statistics in the Debates over Black Mental
Health in the United States, 1840–1900," *Endeavour* 45, no. 1–2 (2021): 100766.

COVER PHOTOGRAPH: "Central State Hospital, Virginia. Camp for Female Consumptives,
1904." From William F. Drewry, *Historical Sketch of the CSH and the Care of the Colored
Insane of Virginia, 1870–1905* (1905). Courtesy of the Library of Virginia, Richmond.

LIBRARY OF CONGRESS CATALOGING-IN-PUBLICATION DATA

Names: Edwards-Grossi, Élodie, author.
Title: Mad with freedom : the political economy of Blackness, insanity, and civil rights in
the U.S. South, 1840–1940 / Élodie Edwards-Grossi.
Description: Baton Rouge : Louisiana State University Press, [2022] | Includes bibliographical
references and index.
Identifiers: LCCN 2022005047 (print) | LCCN 2022005048 (ebook) | ISBN
978-0-8071-7774-7 (cloth) | ISBN 978-0-8071-7865-2 (pdf) | ISBN 978-0-8071-7864-5 (epub)
Subjects: LCSH: African Americans—Mental health—Southern States—History. | African
Americans—Mental health services—Southern States—History. | African Americans—
Southern States—Psychology—History. | Psychiatric Hospitals—Southern States—
History. | Racism in medicine—Southern States—History. | Psychiatry—Southern
States—History. | Racism—Social aspects—Southern States—History. | Mental illness—
Southern States—History.
Classification: LCC RC451.5.B53 E39 2022 (print) | LCC RC451.5.B53 (ebook) |
DDC 362.2/108996075—dc23/eng/20220217
LC record available at https://lccn.loc.gov/2022005047
LC ebook record available at https://lccn.loc.gov/2022005048

TO PAUL AND ALBERTINE

Contents

Acknowledgments

Mad with Freedom began many years ago, in 2013, in Chicago; moved on quite unexpectedly to Los Angeles between 2015 and 2017; navigated to New Orleans between 2017 and 2018; and finally landed in Paris, France, after a short stint in Oxford. This book could not have been produced without the support of my colleagues, friends, and family, as well as the many people I had the fortune to meet during this transatlantic endeavor. I am deeply indebted to Dominique Vidal (URMIS, University of Paris) for his support and encouragement. Likewise, the project would never have gotten under way had it not been for Paul Schor (LARCA, University of Paris), whose advice proved crucial during my first year in Paris. I remember our many discussions on the discipline of being a historian, the tricks of the trade, as it were, and I thank him for his friendship and his continued support over the years.

I was fortunate to have other mentors in France during the early years of the project. I fervently thank the members of the GERMES seminar (URMIS), who provided me with a very helpful network of support and many opportunities for discussion, which came as a welcome refuge from the libraries and archives: Rosane Braud, Marguerite Cognet, Camille Foubert, Olga Gonzalez, Agnès Lainé, Aurélie Racioppi, Maria Teixeira, and Simeng Wang. During graduate school, I met many talented U.S. historians and anthropologists working on race relations in France who guided me at various stages of the project: Jim Cohen, Elisabeth Cunin, Claude-Olivier Doron, Aurélie Godet, Thomas Grillot, Jean-Paul Lallemand-Stempak, Hélène Le Dantec-Lowry, Olivier Richomme, Caroline Rolland-Diamond, Mahamet Timera. I was able to present early drafts of these book chapters at conferences in France, and I am most grateful to Raphaël Gallien, Romain Huret, Alexandre Klein, Aurélia Michel, Delphine Peiretti-Courtis, Emmanuelle Sibeud, and Michel Prum for their critical feedback. I also wish to thank colleagues at the Université de Versailles St-Quentin-en-Yvelines, where I taught for one year, for their support.

I am also indebted to many colleagues at the CAS research center (Université Toulouse Jean Jaurès) for the encouragement and cheer I have received over the last two years, as well as to my colleagues at the IRISSO (Université Paris Dauphine) for their warm welcome and their interest in the project. Thanks are also due to the editorial team at the Presses Universitaires de Rennes, who helped me publish the sister book to *Mad with Freedom*—pertaining to twentieth- and twenty-first-century psychiatric theories and practices, titled *Bad Brains*—in August 2021.

Having spent numerous years as a student, and then as a researcher, in the United States, I am grateful to the many scholars that I have met along the way. At UCLA, I am indebted to Hannah Landecker for her welcome at the Institute for Society and Genetics, as well as Eric Vilain for his help in making my two-year stay in California possible as a visiting researcher with EpiDaPo. The support staff at the ISG helped make the relocation from Paris to Los Angeles as smooth as possible: Anna Avila, Danielle Shenise, Ana Wevill. This book benefited from the wisdom and stimulating conversations I had with Joel Braslow, Soraya de Chadarevian, Marcia Meldrum, and Ted Porter at the Department of History at UCLA, who gave me precious feedback on early versions of the book chapters when I needed it most. In particular, I am grateful for the opportunity to have attended Ted Porter's graduate seminar, where I gained precious insight on historiography. At the ISG, I also benefited from the luminous remarks of Chris Kelty and Aaron Panofsky on early drafts, as well as bibliographical indications. I am also indebted to Joan Donovan, who made my writing days much lighter and with whom I could share my passion for punk music and classic sociology. *Mad with Freedom* would not have been possible without the unfailing support of the French research team at EpiDaPo between 2015 and 2016, who filled my days with helpful advice and good times and kept me energized throughout these Californian years.

I also took *Mad with Freedom* down to Louisiana in 2017 and 2018, where I spent a year as a Fulbright researcher at Tulane University. I am grateful to Kris Lane and Randy Sparks for their warm welcome when I arrived in Tulane's Department of History. My work has benefited from Sparks's seminar and the fruitful conversations we had about early versions of the book chapters. I am also indebted to Tulane faculty members Rosane Adderley, Emily Clark, Kate Edwards, Karissa Haugeberg, and Thomas Klingler for their kind advice and encouragement, as well as to Mark Roudané for his help with the retrieval of archival sources pertaining to his ancestor, Dr. Louis Charles Roudanez. My time in New Orleans slightly overlapped with my affiliated researcher position at the Maison Française, Oxford. I wish to thank director Frédéric Thibault-Starzyk for his welcome.

Public debate was also instrumental in shaping this book, and I must thank the organizers of conferences and seminars both across the Atlantic and across the English Channel, notably at Monmouth University, Princeton University, UCLA, Atlanta (HSS), the University of Liverpool, New Orleans (HSS), Rice University, and the Lapidus Center in New York City, between 2014 and 2021. I am indebted to Chris Willoughby, whom I met in 2016 on my first research trip to Louisiana, and who with remarkable generosity integrated me into the network of U.S. historians working on issues of race and medicine. My many thanks also go to the historians that I met at these conferences, for their friendship and for their excellent comments on my work: Deirdre Cooper Owens, Jim Downs, Urmi Engineer Willoughby, Sharla Fett, Jason Hauser, Rana Hogarth, Bill Horne, Stephen Kenny, and Sean Morey Smith. Thanks also to Rand Dotson and the editorial staff at Louisiana State University Press, who have been most patient and helpful throughout the publication process.

I owe special thanks to those who facilitated the archival research for the manuscript, in particular the archivists at the Library of Congress, the National Archives, the Library of Virginia in Richmond, and the State Archives of North Carolina in Raleigh, who moved heaven and earth to direct me, in record time, to documents relevant to my research. Thanks also to King Davis at UT Austin and Vanessa Jackson for their guidance in the early days of the project. I am indebted to Germain Bienvenu and Amanda K. Hawk, who walked me through the labyrinth of the LSU Libraries Special Collections, and to Mary Holt, at Tulane University, who accompanied me through the depths of the Rudolph Matas Library of the Health Sciences to find old medical notebooks pertaining to my work.

Financial support from a number of institutions enabled me to devote myself fully to the project. The Institut des Sciences Humaines et Sociales (CNRS) offered generous funding that allowed me to spend two years at the Institute for Society and Genetics at UCLA as a visiting graduate researcher. Fulbright France and the Georges Lurcy Charitable and Educational Trust funded this research project over the academic year 2017–2018, which allowed me to be affiliated to the History Department at Tulane University, in

New Orleans. The University of Paris, the URMIS laboratory, the Institut des Amériques, the French Association for American Studies, and NYU Center in Paris all provided support in the form of travel and research grants. Thanks also to Académie des Sciences, Inscriptions et Belles-Lettres de Toulouse, the French Association for American Studies, Fulbright-France, Université PSL (Paris Sciences et Lettres), and Société Française d'Histoire de la Médecine for publicly acknowledging their trust in me by awarding this work their annual prize.

Finally, I would like to express my deepest thanks to my friends and family who have supported me through this long and sometimes winding journey. My fellow graduate students whom I met in the academic institutions I visited provided companionship in cafés, libraries, seminars, and conferences and made my life so much less difficult than it could have been: Iris Clever, Joshua McGuffie, Irene Pasquetto at UCLA; Emmanuel Casajus, Marion Ink, Gabriel Lattanzio, Marion Marchet, Pauline Picot, Tatiana Medvedeva, Aurélie Racioppi in Paris, Marie Alhinho, Chiara Azzaretti, Antoine de Baets, Katherine Sager, Jacqueline Sarro, Olivia Simard in New Orleans. It seems also in order to acknowledge some close personal friends in France and in the U.S. who kept me well amused, well fed, well rested, and ready to head back to seminars and libraries in the morning: Catherine Dixon in Boston; Akanksha Gudiseva, Pilar Martínez-Hidalgo, Marilia Ramos, Till Überrück in Los Angeles; the members of Touchy Coma in Paris; and most warmly Camille Garnon, Laure Jourdan, Hélène Le Cornec, Elodie Nunes, and Lucie Olivieri, who always believed that I could write a book of American history. I wish to thank my family, the Grossis, who gave me time and space to complete this long-term project, and the Edwardses, who opened their homes to me from the start. Most importantly, however, I want to acknowledge my husband, Paul Edwards, for following me on a wild ride across the United States and for his unfailing support. His presence, along with that of our daughter, Albertine, has made my work and life more meaningful.

MAD

WITH

FREEDOM

INTRODUCTION

Anger is better. There is a sense of being in anger. A reality and presence.
An awareness of worth. It is a lovely surging.

—TONI MORRISON, *The Bluest Eye*

In the midst of the 1960s, award-winning novelist James Baldwin campaigned against systemic inequalities and the perpetuation of symbolic and physical violence against Blacks in the United States. In his various speeches and public engagements—one of the most famous being the 1965 debate at the Cambridge Union against William F. Buckley, a conservative commentator and strong defender of racial segregation—Baldwin repeatedly defined the American dream as a far distant utopia for Blacks in this country.[1] The United States had recently experienced a wave of racial violence perpetrated by groups of white supremacists, including members of the Ku Klux Klan. In 1955, Emmett Till, a fourteen-year-old black teenager, had been brutally murdered in the state of Mississippi. The same year, Reverend George Lee, vice president of the Regional Council of Negro Leadership and active member of the NAACP, was assassinated, along with Lamar Smith, a sixty-three-year-old farmer and World War II veteran, both having been actively engaged in encouraging black residents of the Mississippi Delta to exercise their right to vote. In September 1961, Herbert Lee, a black farmer who had participated in campaigns to register Blacks in Mississippi, was murdered by E. H. Hurst, a member of the Mississippi State Assembly. On June 12, 1963, Medgar Evers, one of the field secretaries of the NAACP in Jackson, Mississippi, was assassinated by Byron De La Beckwith, a white supremacist. A black church in Birmingham, Alabama, was bombed on September 15, 1963, leaving several people dead.[2]

Such violent incidents (only a selection of which are presented here) were reported with alarming regularity in the newspapers and weeklies over the 1950s and 1960s, and they made abundantly evident the existence of social and territorial inequalities, as well as systemic racism, affecting the black American population a hundred years after the abolition of slavery. Though racial violence had never disappeared, nor had lynching, this resurgence of violence was without doubt a reaction to the actions of civil rights groups who were pushing for the advancement of black civil rights and desegregation in the South.

In this context, James Baldwin used madness as a metaphor for political resistance, to explain how Blacks could react to systemic violence. "I sometimes feel it to be an absolute miracle that the entire black population of the United States of America has not long ago succumbed to raging paranoia," said Baldwin, linking social inequalities suffered by Blacks in the country to a psychiatric disorder. "Well, I may or may not be bitter, but if I were, I would have good reasons for it," argued Baldwin, explaining that "American blindness, or cowardice," has allowed Blacks "to pretend that life presents no reasons for being bitter," pointing at the invisibilization of black trajectories and suffering in U.S. society.[3]

For Baldwin, Blacks could all have sunk into a state of systemic paranoia, given the social and racist inequalities unfolding in American society and affecting their relationship to the social world. Baldwin's words were framed in direct response to psychiatrists' and psychologists' utilization of the notion of maladjustment to qualify the social behavior of Blacks in the 1960s, at the very time when schizophrenia was diagnosed much more frequently among black Americans than among Whites.[4] Baldwin's choice of the term *paranoia* carried a new meaning, far removed from its use in psychiatry. It did not indicate a medical symptom but instead defined the permanent struggle and the insurrection of Blacks against the oppression they suffered. Furthermore, the unsuitability of Blacks for American society was the product of the racist society in which they lived, which, at the same time, promised them better times ahead, while ever and again reproducing the same social inequalities.[5] Baldwin used this stigmatized identity (maladjustment to society, commonly diagnosed by psychiatrists) to claim that this state was an inherent characteristic of black behavior, indeed a part of their identity, since it was the product of the systemic racism they had suffered for centuries. In sum, the pathologization was in fact the reflection of the racist social, political, and moral order of American society in the 1960s.

Sociologist Erving Goffman theorized that individuals could transform perceived negative characteristics, such as the stigma of maladjustment, into a positive trait when reclaiming their pride and identity. In reversing this stigma, Baldwin was aware that psychiatrists used the term *paranoia* to medicalize behaviors that Baldwin saw as *rational* reactions to racism and systemic poverty. Black activists from Malcolm X to H. Rap Brown to Stokely Carmichael all had been diagnosed with schizophrenia by psychiatric experts commissioned by the FBI, as historian of psychiatry Jonathan Metzl has revealed, thus showing that black political activism was pathologized as mental deviance in the 1960s.[6]

It is precisely from this perspective that this book proposes to unveil the social history of psychiatric theories and practices targeting black patients, from the end of slavery to the early twentieth century, in order to shed light on the systemic medicalization and psychiatrization of the black body in American society. While the 1960s are beyond the scope of this study, there is, in many ways, a cultural and ideological continuity between the pathologization of civil rights and blackness in the twentieth century and in the slavery and post–Civil War eras. Particular attention will be paid to the politicization of science and psychiatric practices, especially with regard to notions of citizenship, responsibility, and civil rights, from the 1840s through the 1930s.

Has there been any significant evolution in the successive categorizations of mental illnesses applied to Blacks in American society since the nineteenth century? Or, to put it another way, were the theories developed in the medical field concerning social maladjustment and mental deviance the result of a psychiatric classification aimed at strengthening the social control of racialized populations? Can certain stereotypes still used today—those, for example, describing black women as particularly "angry" or "aggressive" or even "schizophrenic" when they express strong political opinions—be linked to distinct historical periods remote from our own, such as the nineteenth century, or to periods closer to our own?[7]

The purpose of this book is to provide answers to these questions by studying the evolution of theories relating to mental deviance affecting black bodies specifically and produced by mainly white physicians and psychiatrists in the United States, from the 1840s through the early decades of the twentieth century. To this end, the book examines the political economy of blackness, insanity, and civil rights from the last decades of the slavery era to the first decades of the twentieth century. By "political economy," I refer to the organizing system of values and practices such as those held by southern medical professionals in the nineteenth century, who aimed to create new political meanings and systems of actions relating to the control of black bodies and minds. The notion of political economy is therefore not restricted to the field of economics but also relates to broader historical and sociological concepts that tackle the functions and strategies of individuals who are tied together by professional networks, similar interests, or political opinions.

Drawing on the vast body of historical and sociological works on the long history of racial discrimination in medicine in the United States, and on the construction of a medical apartheid in hospitals in the South since the end of the nineteenth century, my goal has been to write an institutional history of psychiatric spaces that confined black patients, as well as a social history of psychiatric theories and practices that defined the black body as a carrier of specific pathologies. Mixing social history with historical sociology, this book traces the different regimes according to which the notion of blackness was deemed relevant by psychiatrists to naturalize behavioral differences. I maintain that the development of differential psychiatric theories and practices by white doctors to control and cure black patients influenced, in turn, the history of southern political culture during the Jim Crow era in the nineteenth and twentieth centuries, when the "separate but equal" legal principle was extended to all public facilities and transportation, thus enforcing de jure segregation.

Although psychiatry often has been viewed as a discipline that unites a therapeutic motive with a more disciplinary project of social control, as described famously in Michel Foucault's seminal work on psychiatric hospitals and techniques of power, the political history of blackness in psychiatry in the United States, and its intersection with issues of civil rights, marginalization, and medicalization of deviance, has not given rise to many publications.[8] Some groundbreaking books, such as William Stanton's The Leopard's Spots (1960) and Alexander Thomas and Samuel Sillen's Racism and Psychiatry (1972), have paved the way for historians and American studies scholars to look at the organization of medical and psychiatric knowledge in relation to stereotypes of otherness in the United States.[9] American studies scholar Jonathan Metzl's work on the institutionalization of black patients from the early twentieth century onward took a local approach, by looking solely at records of one state hospital in the North, leaving aside the advent of psychiatry in the South.[10]

More recently, works by Dennis Doyle, Gabriel N. Mendes, and Mical Raz have renewed the field of studies on psychiatry, medicine, and blackness by focusing on segregative practices in the twentieth century in northern institutions, but not in southern hospitals.[11] While Doyle and Mendes have tackled the history of psychiatric clinics and hospitals that were located in black ghettoes such as Harlem, Raz has thoughtfully analyzed the advent of psychiatric theories linked to the social control of black bodies and the pathologization of black poverty in the neoliberal age. These works have concentrated on the twentieth century and the advent of northern psychiatry in relation to the treatment of black patients, without focusing on southern institutional history.

As with any work on the history of race and medicine in the United States, this book is indebted to the scholarship of historians who have recently revisited the history of health and medicine on southern plantations, in the Atlantic World, and in the context of colonial empires, such as Manuella Meyer's work on psychiatry in Brazil in the nineteenth and twentieth centuries, Jim Downs's monograph about the rise of administrative medical classifications in the context of slavery and the British Empire, and Delphine Peiretti-Courtis's book about the French colonial state and medicine.[12] For example, Sharla Fett and Londa Schiebinger examined how enslaved people engaged in their own set of healing practices, competing directly with white medical practices that reified black bodies.[13] Other scholars, such as Stephen C. Kenny, Deirdre Cooper Owens, Rana Hogarth, Vincent Woodard, and Daina Ramey Berry, have shown how white physicians appropriated and abused enslaved bodies in order to advance scientific knowledge in the plantation South.[14]

While some works have also tackled specific racialized theories on black behavior, focusing on controversial medical figures such as Samuel Cartwright or James Babcock, no study currently exists on how these physicians' models contributed to the long-term evolution of theories on insanity and blackness in the United States.[15] Other works have dealt with medicine and race in the postbellum era in the South. Jim Downs's monograph *Sick from Freedom* tells the largely unknown story of how many formerly enslaved people died at the time of their newfound freedom, narrating the harsh biomedical realities that freed slaves had to deal with during and after the Civil War, while Gretchen Long's monograph examines black individuals' resistance and struggles to obtain medical care in the context of Jim Crow.[16] Focusing on sterilization laws and eugenics in Virginia after the 1920s, Pippa Holloway explores the history of mental institutions in the state and how black patients were treated as a sexual danger in the context of social and political anxiety over interracial relationships and "passing."[17]

Although this scholarship has, overall, produced a dynamic image of medical practices to control black bodies, ranging from racialized treatments to sterilization in various southern states, it did not aim to explore the evolution of politically charged medical theories on insanity after the 1860s and the building of what might be called a "medical apartheid" in southern hospitals after emancipation.[18] Furthermore, works focusing either on the antebellum plantations, on the postbellum era, or solely on the 1920s onward also tend to fracture the continuities that might exist in medical theories between the 1840s and the early twentieth century.

Other books have recently considered the history of southern asylums for Blacks in the South, such as Mab Segrest's, Wendy Gonaver's, and Martin Summers's recent studies on race and madness in the nineteenth century and early twentieth century, in Georgia, Virginia, and Washington, DC, respectively.[19] Segrest's book tackles the specific history of the Milledgeville asylum in Georgia from the 1840s until the 1940s and draws a parallel between this institution and Nazi concentration camps.[20] Gonaver's scholarship recounts the history of the gradual internment of black patients within the Eastern Lunatic Asylum in Williamsburg, Virginia, from the 1840s until 1880, and also covers the opening in the 1870s of the Central Lunatic Asylum at Petersburg, Virginia, one of the first institutions in the United States dedicated to black patients.

These two books provide thoughtful vignettes that show how the treatment of black patients was organized in these local Virginia and Georgia institutions, but they do not necessarily discuss the broader southern regional dynamics at stake in the institutionalization of black patients categorized as mentally ill in the nineteenth and early twentieth centuries. Gonaver's study focuses solely on the very beginnings of today's Central State Hospital at Petersburg, and deals in a thoughtful way with the use of mechanical restraints on patients at this institution and with how physicians at the hospital used religion as a variable to measure the degree of "excitement" of black patients. Considering that the Petersburg facility operated as a psychiatric institution for Blacks only until the 1960s, its history in the early twentieth century could be further expanded. Finally, Martin Summers's work on St. Elizabeths Hospital in Washington, DC, has unveiled the patterns of racialization in this segregated federal institution, from its foundation and into the twentieth century.

Although the present book is undoubtedly in line with these previous works of scholarship on race and madness in the nineteenth century, it expands upon this topic by concentrating on race, civil rights, and the politicization of madness through forced labor, a conjunction that has been overlooked in the historiography. Consequently, it fills a historiographical void in the evolution of the political history of madness and blackness in the U.S. South. Drawing on the large body of historical and sociological work dedicated to the long history of medical discrimination and race, I contend that the history of the rise of racialized psychiatric theories in the early nineteenth century has outgrown the parameters of the history of slavery, as well as the history of science, by impacting the post-emancipation era. The development of racial medicine and theories on black behavior between 1840 and 1940 not only produced biodeterminist concepts of race but also informed notions of citizenship and civil rights, as psychiatry metamorphosed into a truly political science.

Indeed, white physicians, using their scientific authority and public visibility, were simultaneously *politicizing* medical theories and *medicalizing* political deviance. They often pathologized the behaviors of their black patients, whom they saw as indocile, as too political, or as prone to sexual deviance, and chose to treat these behaviors through forced labor as a way to tame black masculinity and political resistance to the southern social order.[21] They often naturalized the links between madness and freedom, arguing that the latter caused changes in behavior after 1865, and thus participated in a new political economy of psychiatric theories in the nineteenth century around forced labor and race.

The book's focus on the evolution of racial epidemiologies in the nineteenth and early twentieth centuries also brings attention to the understudied topic of the conflict between the internationalization of science and the local concepts and practices adopted by physicians. Consequently, I aim to reveal the discontinuities and continuities between proto-psychiatric theories in the nineteenth century and the spread of racist scientific frameworks later on, in the early twentieth century, while interrogating the traditional break between the antebellum and postbellum periods. The book will therefore combine a reflection on the history of racialized social control in psychiatry in the United States with the history of racialized pathologies, while also contributing to a history of the medical profession and segregated hospitals.

These fields of study (history of science, history of medicine, history of psychiatry, black history, history of the U.S. South, and historical sociology), although they sometimes deal with related subjects, are considerably fragmented.[22] For example, works focusing on the history of race and medicine, and which deal specifically with plantations in the antebellum South, or with the twentieth century, tend to break the continuities that could exist in medical theories between the 1840s and the early twentieth century. It is also to be noted that this historical research has mainly focused on controversial medical figures such as Samuel Cartwright or Marion J. Sims, or on particular events such as the medical experiments at Tuskegee, and has not given an account of the historical evolution of the racialist health care system as a whole over time. Consequently, I turn the spotlight away from singular historical events such as the Tuskegee affair, which is already profusely documented, or from eugenics practices, which tend to obscure the invisible, yet omnipresent, everyday practices of racialized science: the classifications adopted by psychiatrists, the systematic and routine treatments imposed on patients, and the strategic positioning of doctors in relation to the notion of race. Instead, this book explores a history of medicine that has little to do with individual medical figures but much to do with everyday practices structured by institutional racism.

The choice of the period to be covered, from the 1840s through the 1930s, was determined by several parameters. First, the 1840s marked the publication of the first medical journals devoted exclusively to theories of insanity in the United States, including the *American Journal of Insanity*. Starting with this period was a way of taking into account the beginnings of what could be called proto-psychiatry, at the very time when many asylums were opened throughout America. In the United States before the 1840s, insanity was generally considered to be a disease mostly affecting Whites, based on several factors that will be analyzed in chapter 1. Second, the first theories on the madness of Blacks emerged during the 1840s, in both the South and the North, under the impulse of the first reactions to the statistics of the 1840 census, as will be discussed in chapter 2. The book stops after the 1930s, which is the decade during which northern mental health institutions started to institutionalize black patients, after the Great Migration.[23]

Out of the hundred or so asylums and state hospitals that opened in the Jim Crow South to treat black mentally ill populations, only specific institutions scattered across the U.S. South—in Virginia, Louisiana, and North Carolina—as well as in Washington, DC, are under scrutiny here. There are two main reasons for this choice. First, these institutions offer well-preserved archival holdings. Second, each was situated in a different southern state, thus making it possible to draw a more global and comparative portrait of the different situations that existed for Blacks in psychiatric hospitals in the South.[24] Some of these institutions, including the Central Lunatic Asylum in Petersburg, Virginia (called the Central State Hospital after the 1890s; see figures 1 and 2), and the Eastern North Carolina Insane Asylum (the State Hospital at Goldsboro), were exclusively for black patients, while others, such as the Central Louisiana State Hospital in Pineville, Louisiana (originally known as the Louisiana Hospital for the Insane), treated both black and white patients in separate wards.

It is worth noting that these hospitals have not previously been studied in comparison with each other, but only separately. While some of them (especially the Central State Hospital in Virginia, though only up to the 1880s, and St. Elizabeths Hospital in Washington, DC) have been mentioned in previous articles or books, writing about these institutions reveals the differences and nuances in therapeutic practices in each state while painting a broader picture of southern U.S. asylums, which is very much needed and has not yet been provided. Studying the archives of various southern asylums and hospitals that

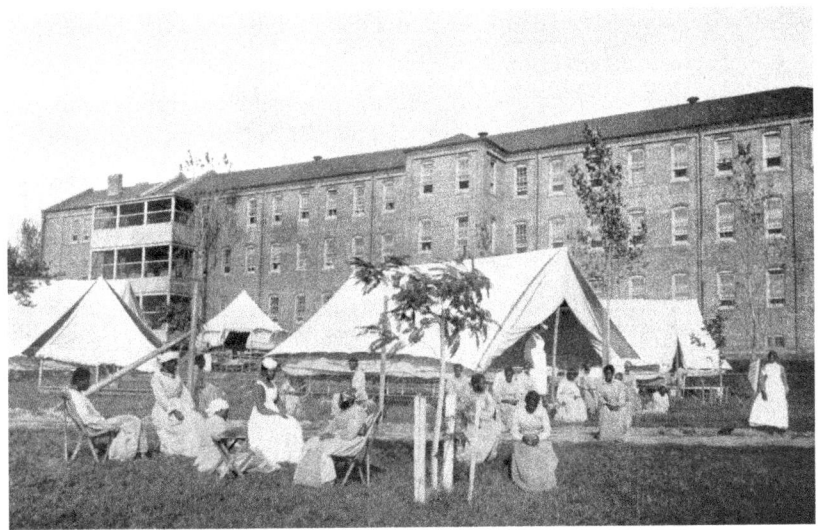

FIGURE 1. "Central State Hospital, Virginia. Camp for Female Consumptives, 1904." From William F. Drewry, *Historical Sketch of the CSH and the Care of the Colored Insane of Virginia, 1870–1905* (1905).

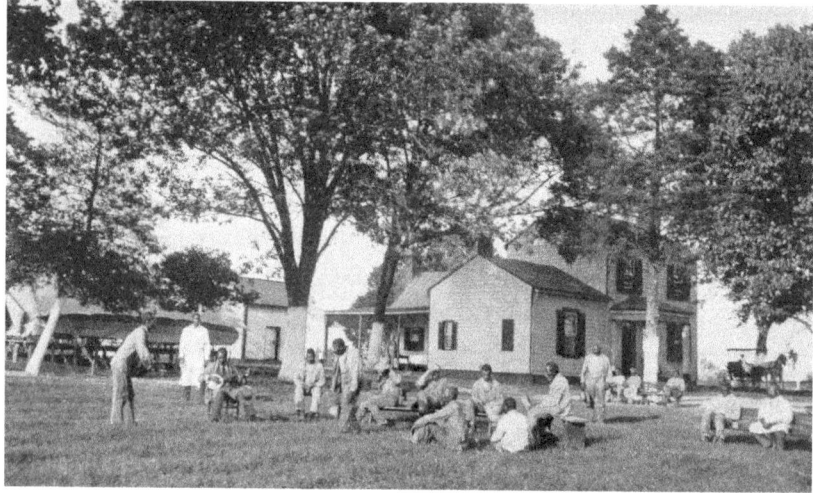

FIGURE 2. "Ashleigh Grange Colony, Central State Hospital, Virginia, Petersburg."
From William F. Drewry, *Historical Sketch of the CSH and the Care of the Colored Insane of Virginia, 1870–1905* (1905).

hosted black patients during the nineteenth century unveils the normalization of psychiatric spaces, their conditioning, and their internal functioning in relation to the racial dividing line, across the southern states. Understanding the context of creation of these institutions, their differences, and their similarities, through the study of various historical vignettes, as well as examining the theories and practices developed by physicians, offers a broader portrait of racialized psychiatric treatments in the southern states from the 1840s through the 1930s. Moreover, some of the institutions or archival collections examined here, including the institutions in Goldsboro and Pineville, have seldom been studied.

The book draws on the writings of famous historical figures, such as Dorothea Dix and Samuel Cartwright, who have of course been explored in other publications. But it also examines some overlooked sources in the historiography, such as the writings of physicians Judson B. Andrews, Robert F. Baldwin, Stanford Emerson Chaillé, Daniel Burr Conrad, Theodore Diller, Joseph Jones, W. C. Linville, J. D. Roberts, Martin Scott, J. W. Vick, A. H. Witmer, and Louis Charles Roudanez, one of the only black doctors in Louisiana in the 1860s. The book also relies on the archives of the Medical College of Louisiana, one of the first medical schools in the South that trained white doctors in the treatment of black bodies in the nineteenth century. The writings of physicians such as Stanford Emerson Chaillé and Joseph Jones, both of whom were professors in this institution, will therefore be discussed.

The book examines often overlooked archival records from both Anglophone and Francophone sources, especially those relating to the history of Louisiana. Overall, *Mad with Freedom* displays a wide range of sources: personal papers of physicians and activists, oral histories, patients' testimonies, municipal archives, state archives, federal archives, and newspapers.[25]

The last chapter will also analyze the evolution of racial classifications in southern asylums from the late nineteenth century through the 1930s, as psychoanalytic theories took over some of the previous nosological categories in place in the 1870s and 1880s. The psychoanalytic theories developed by physicians at St. Elizabeths Hospital will also be examined in the context of transnational circulations between Europe and the United States.

The book thus aims to analyze the political economy of psychiatric treatment in the South by examining local medical networks, starting from the theories developed in medical schools in the South; the circulation of articles published in leading medical journals regularly consulted by doctors; and hospital practice from the 1840s through the 1930s. Although the book focuses mostly on the theories and institutional practices of white physicians treating black patients, some chapters also attempt to reconstruct the black patients' strategies of resistance to moral therapies, in an attempt to shift the focus away from medical theorists. Even if most of their names and voices have been lost, the book attempts to reclaim these patients' place in history. However, I was limited by the historical sources to be found in the archives; most often, only the voices of white physicians were present in the records, while the patients' voices, as well as their individual thoughts and actions, have been erased from the institutional reports and physicians' papers. The silence left by the erasure of these patients' voices nonetheless informs us about the existing power dynamics at stake in the southern asylums, as sites of alienation and repression.

I embrace an activist vision of history in its propensity to enter into contact with more contemporary themes. Likewise, it did not seem desirable to write a story from above. Instead, I have chosen to combine social history with sociology, with the desire to remain open to different audiences for the research themes studied and to foster the development of research that is fully engaged with everyday life, providing actors in the social world with the critical tools and reflective strategies necessary for the conduct of struggles and the questioning of the status quo. Throughout this book, I have thus attempted a "public social history," to use a term derived from public sociology, as theorized by Michael Burawoy, to define the sociological practice made available to actors in civil society.[26]

The first chapter covers the years 1840 to 1860, a period that corresponds to the emergence of the first theories on the madness of enslaved people and free people of color, shortly after the creation of the *American Journal of Insanity*, which delimited a new field of study for American physicians who published about mental disorders, who were then still not unified as a profession. Chapter 1 is an opportunity to write a sociohistory of the invention of diagnoses of madness and other behavioral disorders as they were applied to the black population in the southern states before the Civil War. This chapter focuses on the early theories about enslaved people and their so-called behavioral problems, as developed by the doctors of the Medical College of Louisiana in New Orleans (founded in 1834 and one of the first medical institutions in the South) and by physicians from the same region such as Samuel Cartwright. Although Cartwright's theories are well known, I focus on showing how those theories were disseminated in the South, both in medical and political circles, and how they forged a connection between race, madness, and moral treatment such as forced labor. These theories on forced labor would later be reused by medical superintendents in racially segregated asylums and in asylums for Blacks in the post–Civil War era to politicize madness, as shown in chapters 3 and 4.

In connection to these theoretical frameworks, chapter 1 also analyzes the various debates that from the 1840s onward split the southern medical field over the internment of enslaved people in institutions such as the Eastern Lunatic Asylum in Virginia, one of the very first southern institutions to intern black patients before the Civil War. The chapter builds upon recent findings concerning the Eastern Lunatic Asylum, but it also highlights new aspects of the history of this institution and the admission of free Blacks prior to 1841, as well as the history of racial integration in the institution. Although this institution's medical superintendent pushed for reformist policies such as racial integration within the asylum, chapter 1 notes that such policies constituted an exception in the 1840s. This departs from the historiography, which often has presented this institution as a case that could be generalized. Thus, this chapter advances another important argument: instead of focusing solely on local histories, it shows how the South can be constructed as a somewhat homogenous medical and political landscape when dealing with race and madness. Throughout the antebellum period, the diagnosis of madness among black populations was not systematized, due to the reluctance of enslavers to declare enslaved people as "mentally ill" and therefore not fit for labor.

The second chapter tells the story of the results of the 1840 census with regard to the number of black and white "lunatics" in the northern states and how these results shaped southern physicians' understanding of free Blacks' madness as a public and political problem at the federal level. Southern medical and political circles were eager to seize on these statistics to attest to the dangerousness of free Blacks, whose very freedom was supposed to have been the cause of their madness. Consequently, this chapter analyzes how the circulation of these figures, though they were disproven, facilitated the promotion of the first theories of madness affecting black populations in the United States, and of theories naturalizing the black body between 1840 and 1890, in a context marked by sectionalist tensions between the North and the South. This chapter therefore shows that the gradual medicalization of black bodies followed the local debates on the civil rights of Blacks and their potential emancipation.

The chapter also highlights the stubbornness of southern physicians and southern commentators, who continued to refer to the 1840 census returns, or to follow-up results, to explain that slavery was a positive good, despite the figures having been proved erroneous by various commentators from the North or from abroad. Consequently, these theories on blackness, insanity, and freedom also circulated in the North, in places like Detroit and New York, as well as abroad, where U.S. census returns were discussed and bitterly criticized by European naturalist Ramón de la Sagra. This discussion makes it possible to decenter previous discussions about the 1840 census, previously limited to the United States, by looking at the perspective of an outsider such as de la Sagra and the different arguments he brought to the table to denaturalize the links between madness and race that southern physicians had attempted to push forward.

The chapter also discusses James McCune Smith, one of the first black doctors living in New York at the time, and Zion Church's black community and their criticisms of the 1840 census. Their perspectives show that although black ministers and the black community engaged in the debates concerning the interpretation of the census, those black voices often have been erased and not commented upon in previous scholarship, which has focused on the denunciation of the statistical results by northern white physicians such as Edward Jarvis. Consequently, this chapter deals with black agency and the possibility of black resistance to the medical and political apparatuses at the time.

Chapter 3 recounts the opening of the first asylums and hospitals for black patients in Virginia, North Carolina, and Louisiana during and after Reconstruction, a period that marks the end of the southern regime. Although some hospitals, including the Eastern Lunatic Asylum in Virginia, had opened their doors to some black patients in the 1840s and later, few specific and systematic prerogatives had been issued by southern legislators between 1840 and 1870 to accommodate the mentally ill black population in the South. This chapter explores the context and debates behind the opening of these hospitals in three different states, including similarities among them, such as the systematic reluctance of Whites to finance a system of public assistance for Blacks until the 1910s.

In addition, it looks at the pathologization of emancipation and blackness following the Civil War, which has been overlooked in the historiography. The new social status that enslaved people gained after 1865—they were now considered freedmen and freedwomen and enjoyed new civil rights—was pathologized by southern physicians, who used their medical authority to diagnose insanity in the free black population in unprecedented numbers. Chapter 3 builds on chapter 2, which focuses on the use of insanity statistics by southern physicians who wished to show that insanity was more prevalent among free Blacks than among the enslaved population in the pre–Civil War era. Chapter 3 unveils how these arguments linking madness to emancipation were still used by southern physicians in those asylums in the post–Civil War era.

Using photographs taken in various southern institutions, this chapter also looks at the overcrowding in those institutions after the 1870s and the relationships between local law enforcement and the asylum staff when it came to finding room for the patients, thus revealing the carceral character of these institutions. The chapter also introduces new findings about the dire financial situation of all-black hospitals compared to white institutions in those states. Building on personal writings by physicians about the functioning of the asylums, the chapter shows the punitive nature and poor material conditions of the asylums for black patients in three southern states.

Moving on to the 1870s through the 1930s, chapter 4 examines how south-

ern physicians organized differential therapeutic treatments to cure black patients in the state hospitals in Virginia, North Carolina, South Carolina, and
Louisiana, while pathologizing political emancipation and naturalizing their
black patients' capacity to work in a docile way. Examining the organization
of distinct racialized work spaces specific to black patients provides examples
of the white physicians' efforts to view physical labor as a curative tool for returning freedmen and freedwomen to sanity by bringing them back to what
was seen as the "natural" laboring condition of enslaved people.

This chapter also shows how the work spaces in segregated asylums and
hospitals were organized along the lines of race and gender. In the Central Louisiana State Hospital in Pineville, across the Red River from the larger city of
Alexandria, white and black men and women were assigned various racialized
and gendered tasks that were supposed to cure and discipline their bodies,
as two faces of the same coin. The photographs reproduced here, which can
be compared with nineteenth-century iconography depicting enslaved black
laborers in the fields, furnish new analytical tools for examining forced labor
and the treatment of madness among black populations through docility and
physical punishment. The chapter also looks at black agency and local, system-
ized resistance to the rigid, institutional organization of labor.

Beyond reconstructing the history of these separate work spaces, chapter
4 deals with the epidemiological categories physicians in institutions in North
Carolina, Virginia, and Louisiana used to treat black and white patients differently, with a strong focus on their discourses about emancipation as a cause
of insanity. This chapter is therefore closely connected to chapter 1 (on the
theories of docility and forced labor in the 1850s), chapter 2 (on the theories
of madness and freedom), and chapter 3 (on forced labor and the asylums as
sites of social control).

One of the contributions of this chapter is to highlight the history of the
categories "political excitement" and "change of life," which after 1865 were
used in southern institutions to pathologize black patients' political activism and, more broadly, their emancipation from slavery. It also discusses the
creation and uses of these overtly politicized nosologies in connection with
race and insanity by physicians such as Judson B. Andrews, Stanford Emerson
Chaillé, Daniel Burr Conrad, Theodore Diller, Joseph Jones, and A. H. Witmer,
whose writings have seldom been commented upon. These writings span from
the 1850s to the 1930s and show how the theorization of emancipation and in-

sanity evolved from the pre–Civil War context to the post–Civil War context in the North and in the South. The chapter also retraces the history of these theories about madness and politics by paying attention to similar categories in the United States and in Europe in moments of political turmoil, such as during the Paris Commune. The theories relating blackness to labor in state asylums, developed by white physicians in North Carolina, Louisiana, and Virginia, offer a striking example of the naturalization of black bodies and indicate the rise of new medical theories linking power, white authority, and the treatment of madness in the post-emancipation era and after the end of Reconstruction.

Finally, chapter 5 offers an analysis of the new pathologies and causes of madness detected by white physicians and psychiatrists, specifically among the black population in segregated hospitals in these three states, from the 1870s through the 1930s. The first part of the chapter looks at the circulation and use in southern medical spaces of local classification categories of "political excitement," which were used to count and class particular cases of insanity affecting Blacks, at a time when new categories were being adopted by the international community, especially in the 1890s and 1900s. The chapter first looks closely at the way in which psychiatrists built essentialist categorizations for groups of populations that they saw as distinct from an epidemiological standpoint and which they labeled as "mulattoes," "Africans," and "American Blacks." By naturalizing these categorizations, they attributed different symbolic meanings to such categories, in the context of discussing sexual deviance and at a time when "passing" and interracial relationships were especially taboo in the South.

The second part of the chapter then examines the psychiatrization of political and sexual deviance by focusing on the rise of psychoanalytic theories that classified black bodies, after psychoanalysis became a popular new field in the 1910s in the United States. The first volumes of the *Psychoanalytic Review* were published in 1913, four years after Sigmund Freud's first visit to the United States. Building upon Summers's previous work on the physicians at St. Elizabeths Hospital, whose writings were deeply influenced by psychoanalytic frameworks, this chapter demonstrates the influence of European psychoanalysts such as Freud and Alfred Adler on this new type of racialist writings. Southern physicians imported their theories on dreams, wish fulfillment, and the inferiority complex—which made no mention of race—and adapted them to the local, segregated context of the U.S. South. The chapter closely examines specific nosologies inspired by Adler's theoretical framework and analyzes the shaping of the "color complex," a term coined and used by Mary O' Malley and John Lind, two physicians in Washington, DC, to pathologize their female and male patients in the early 1920s.

Furthermore, this adaptation of psychoanalytic theories to the southern context highlights a paradox: while black patients were understood to be epidemiologically different from white patients—black patients being placed in separate medical institutions and subject to research that highlighted supposed biological differences between Whites and Blacks—these same patients were no longer thought to be radically different, from an epidemiological point of view, when the opportunity arose for doctors to conduct medical experiments on black bodies for the purpose, openly admitted, of advancing a so-called universalist science. This last chapter therefore investigates the tensions that existed between, on the one hand, the international standardization of science as an ongoing process and, on the other, the local epidemiologies pertaining to the black population.

1

THE "SANE SLAVES"

Theories about Madness and Blackness, 1800–1860

The medicine I remember was castor oil and dogwood and cherry bark,
which they put in whiskey and give you. They give you this to keep your blood
good. Dogwood will bitter your blood; it good medicine, I know.

—AMY PERRY, eighty-two years old, interviewed in May 1937,
in Belinda Hurmence, *Before Freedom*

I n 1847, Dorothea Dix penned a letter to the senators of the state of Tennessee to convince them to back her project to open an asylum for the care of
mentally ill people in their state.[1] A passionate social reformer who advocated for the cure of the indigent mentally ill in the 1840s, Dix had argued for a
number of years for the creation of asylums throughout the United States and
was widely recognized by her peers for her activist work. She grew up in New
England and had been instrumental in the opening of an asylum in Massachusetts in 1843 and in New Jersey in 1844, and she would be similarly successful in
the states of North Carolina, Louisiana, Pennsylvania, and Illinois in the 1850s.[2]
Dix's writings were largely inspired by the works of famous physicians such as
Philippe Pinel in France; Jean-Étienne Dominique Esquirol, Pinel's student at
the Salpêtrière; the Quaker William Tuke in England; and Vincenzo Chiarugi
in Italy. All of them denounced the appalling conditions in which mentally ill
people lived in their respective countries during the first half of the nineteenth
century.[3]

Dix pleaded in front of the legislators in Tennessee, "I ask to lay before
you, briefly and distinctly, the necessities and claims of a numerous, and unfortunately an increasing class of your fellow citizens—I refer to the Insanes

of this State; the various distresses of whose various condition can be fully appreciated only by those who have witnessed their miseries." She painted a dark picture of these diseased individuals, whom she depicted as "pining in cells and dungeons, pent in log cabins, bound with ropes, restrained by leathern throngs, burdened with chains—now wandering at large, alone and neglected, endangering the security of property, often inimical to human life; and now thrust into cells, into pens of wretched cabins, excluded from the fair light of heaven, from social and healing influences—cast out, cast off." Overall, Dix preached the idea that state institutions for the mentally ill could put their patients on the path of moral salvation and redemption while giving them a place of their own, far away from the prison walls.

Although Dix argued in favor of the opening of asylums—which she depicted as institutions symbolizing the epitome of benevolence and advanced medicine at the time—she nevertheless drew up a rigid classification when it came to referencing patients as members of different classes and races. To her, patients from different races should be treated separately, despite the universalist pretensions of her exposé, in which she exhorted the Tennessee legislators to support the opening of a public institution for the mentally ill: "The Negro and the Indian rarely become subject to the malady of insanity, as neither do the uncivilized tribes and clans of European Russia and Asia. Insanity is the malady of civilized and cultivated life, and sections and communities whose nervous energies are most roused and nourished."[4]

Dix's efforts to explain that Indians and Blacks were unable to suffer from mental diseases can be understood as a direct strategy to tone down the relative cost of a public asylum in the state of Tennessee. Indeed, since she was addressing the senators of Tennessee, a state with a considerable number of Blacks and Native Americans in its population at the time, Dix presumably wanted to relativize the overall cost of this new institution by suggesting that these racialized populations within asylum walls would never be a financial burden to the state.[5] Dix's line of argument sought to convince the all-white legislators that her asylum project would not trigger the use of white taxpayers' money to fund racialized patients' welfare. Beyond these financial preoccupations, Dix's correlation between a supposed lack of civilization and an absence of episodes of madness among black populations exemplifies the types of moral and medical discourses that circulated widely in the United States when it came to matters of race and madness.

Here, therefore, I analyze whether physicians and legislators alike saw racialized bodies, and especially the bodies of free people of color or enslaved people, as capable of experiencing madness and thus eligible for internment in public institutions in southern states during the antebellum period. What were the political and moral underpinnings evoked by doctors and medical men in the country to conceptualize madness as an all-white disease and burden?

The first chapter presents the social history of medical diagnoses relating to madness and other behavioral disorders among the black population in the southern states before the Civil War, focusing on the early theories about enslaved people and their behavioral problems that have been overlooked in the historiography about race and madness in the slavery era. These theories were developed by doctors such as Samuel Cartwright and were disseminated through his network of influences in Louisiana. These doctors solidified the interwoven arguments on race, docility, and forced labor to naturalize the living conditions of enslaved people on plantations in the pre–Civil War era, which was a period of drastic economic and demographic changes in the South. Those changes would help shape the political moment in which the ideas of Cartwright and other racialist physicians developed.

From the 1810s to the 1850s, the Second Middle Passage—the forced relocation of enslaved peoples from the upper South to the lower South of the United States to accommodate the spread of the cotton industry from 1790 until 1861—combined with the impact of the Indian Removal Act, transformed the cotton regions of the Deep South into one of the largest and richest slave societies in history.[6] In May 1830, the U.S. House of Representatives passed the Indian Removal Act, opening more cheap land for settlement in the West, which was needed by enslavers to strengthen their economic model in these new territories.[7] Highlighting the rise of these racialist theories in this specific historical context helps to show the extent to which Cartwright was a product of the political economy of this time and how his theories on insanity developed in the context of debates and sectionalist tensions over the Fugitive Slave Act of 1850.

This chapter also aims to analyze the various debates about the internment of enslaved people that split the southern medical field from the 1840s onward in institutions such as the Eastern Lunatic Asylum in Virginia, which was one of the first southern institutions to intern black patients before the Civil War. While this institution has been thoughtfully studied by historian Wendy

Gonaver in her 2019 book, which focuses solely on the situation in the state of Virginia, and more specifically on the Eastern Lunatic Asylum, it remains nonetheless essential to extend her analysis on race and the treatment of insanity before the Civil War. The greater part of the southern medical profession first considered enslaved people's internment as an inadequate measure, preferring punishment and incarceration to redemption, before embracing moral treatment and forced labor in asylums as potential techniques of cure and restraint that could be applied to freed black bodies in the post–Civil War era. My analysis here is also the start of a broader depiction of the southern medical apparatus regarding race, moral treatment, and madness after the 1840s and the birth of modern asylums in Virginia, North Carolina, and Louisiana, to show how these three states responded to each other in their adoption of theories and practices, in different locations and at different times.

From the beginning of the nineteenth century onward, physicians constructed a specific ontology of madness when it came to discussing Blacks' metabolism, which they constructed as biologically distinct. The symbiosis between madness and blackness in the United States goes back to a literature that emerged at the beginning of the nineteenth century and defined the intellectual and moral capacities of each race.[8] Benjamin Rush, often described as the father of psychiatry in the United States, was one of the first doctors to attribute specific mental disorders to enslaved people. In the early 1800s, he reported that mental illnesses came primarily from environmental rather than hereditary causes. Rush had, in particular, developed a theory concerning the preponderance of certain diseases among Blacks, and he had devoted a section of his notes in his scrapbooks to what he called the "peculiar diseases of Negroes," coming just after the section in which he detailed diseases specific to children and women.

Rush explained in chapter 6 of his lecture notes that Blacks were particularly susceptible to jaw infections and that he had treated them for eating "putrid flesh" as well as "insect eggs."[9] For Rush, such eating disorders were a well-known form of irrationality. A few years later, in 1812, in his book *Medical Inquiries and Observations upon the Diseases of the Mind,* Rush would recount that this particular form of madness had developed among enslaved Blacks "soon after they enter the toils of perpetual slavery in the West Indies."[10] According to Rush, who was himself a northerner and an abolitionist, this eating disorder would arise as the result of the deprivation of liberty of black men and women, who aimed to protest enslavement by ingesting dangerous materials. Rush is also famous for having stated that the darker color of enslaved people's skin was due to a form of leprosy.[11] To him, this different complexion resulted in episodes of delirium in enslaved people, a result of the stigma suffered by those excluded from society and dominated by white power.[12]

Rush therefore theorized that these various forms of madness (the eating disorder, and the reaction to having a dark complexion in a white hegemonic society) were afflictions that would arise as a form of enslaved people's social protest against enslavers. All in all, one can find in Rush's theories, dating from the beginning of the nineteenth century, the mark of monogenism, a scientific current defended notably by the northern pastor Samuel Stanhope Smith, who sought to demonstrate that all men belonged to a single human race, with physical appearance varying according to the degree of adaptation to climate.[13]

There were, however, other theories at the beginning of the nineteenth century that proposed a diametrically opposed reading of the mental health of Blacks. These writings insisted on the supposed "primitivism" of their minds, which was seen, in a way, as protecting them from insanity. As an example of this, one may recall Dorothea Dix's statement discussed earlier. According to Dix, in the 1840s, enslaved or Native American peoples were too primitive to be able to feel the complex emotions that would provoke episodes of madness. This medical theory was taken for granted by some physicians and naturalists, for whom Blacks were predisposed to not suffer from mental diseases. Its source was racial science, which attributed intelligence and mental abilities to the different subgroups of the human population.

In the 1820s and 1830s, Samuel G. Morton, a physician from Philadelphia, set out to measure different human skulls by comparing their cranial capacities and then classifying them into distinct population groups.[14] This classification led him to develop a theory in racial physical anthropology and to become one of the pioneers of the discipline, publishing *Crania Americana: or, a Comparative View of the Skulls of Various Aboriginal Nations of North and South America*, among other works. Moreover, Morton was a fervent defender of polygenism and theorized that the different races were from different species with separate origins.[15] Influenced by phrenology, a discipline based on the measurement of the skull as an indicator of moral and physical qualities, he boasted that he could identify the racial origins of any skull by measuring it, as he had drawn up tables based on the measurements he had made on different races previously identified as such. Morton believed that the cranial capacity of Europeans was by far the highest human cranial capacity; then came populations he classified as Chinese, Southeast Asians, and Polynesians; then American Indians; and finally Australian Aborigines and Africans. The skull measurements made by Morton were quoted to support the theory of primitivism of black minds, with the cranial statistics being presented as material proof of a lack of intelligence.

These pseudoscientific theories alleging the primitivism of black brains were also rooted in the writings of Thomas Jefferson, published some sixty years earlier. Over several pages of his famous memoir *Notes on the State of Virginia,* Jefferson discussed what he viewed as the "lack of rationality" of Blacks, claiming that their existence appeared "to participate more of sensation than reflection." In an effort to prove that Blacks were mentally inferior to Whites, Jefferson wrote, "Comparing them by their faculties of memory, reason, and imagination, it appears to me, that in memory they are equal to the whites; in reason much inferior, as I think one could scarcely be found capable of tracing and comprehending the investigations of Euclid; and that in imagination they are dull, tasteless, and anomalous."[16]

The emergence of these successive theories linking intellectual capacities such as reason or imagination with race underlines the paradoxical character of madness as it was then conceived and diagnosed by white physicians in the late eighteenth and early nineteenth centuries. Madness, thought of as a most virulent form of pathology, was seen as the mark of a strong emotional complexity and thus represented a capacity for humanity and modernity, from which Blacks were a fortiori excluded. In the first half of the nineteenth century, the absence of madness among black populations in medical diagnoses and theory can be read as a reflection of the naturalized moral, political, and social order that the doctors wished to preserve.

It was not until the early 1850s that articles mentioning cases of madness affecting black populations started to be published in medical journals, mostly in the South. A close inspection of one of the oldest American medical journals, the *Boston Medical and Surgical Journal,* which had been published since 1812 by the Massachusetts Medical Society (under the title *New England Journal of Medicine, Surgery and Collateral Branches of Science*), reveals the presence of articles dealing with madness from the 1810s up to the 1840s, but none specifically mentioning the existence of madness among Blacks.[17] Some of the articles published between 1820 and 1840 discussed other diseases particularly affecting black men and women; yellow fever, smallpox, measles, abdominal dropsy, hydrothorax, tuberculosis, cataracts, ulcers, toothache, and conditions such as alcoholism are listed as ailments affecting this population, composed mostly of enslaved people.[18] Thus, while in the antebellum South enslaved people were the subjects of medical classifications, madness was not taken into account by southern physicians until the 1850s.[19] What then was at stake for such a radical theoretical upheaval to have taken place?

One of the most influential instigators of the change in perspective was Samuel Adolphus Cartwright (1793–1863), a southern physician who was born in Fairfax County, Virginia, and who later practiced medicine in Huntsville, Alabama, and Natchez, Mississippi, before relocating to New Orleans in his later years.[20] A famous polygenist, rejecting the idea that the black and white "races" had common origins, Cartwright had been educated at Transylvania University in Kentucky.[21] By the early 1850s he had chosen to settle in New Orleans, where the Medical College of Louisiana, one of the first southern medical schools, was founded.

Cartwright's theories have been discussed in recent publications, such as historian Christopher D. E. Willoughby's 2018 article, Steven M. Stowe's 2004 book, and Stephen C. Kenny's 2013 and 2016 articles. They have also been commented upon in Eugene D. Genovese's classic *Roll, Jordan, Roll: The World the Slaves Made* as well as in John S. Haller Jr's 1972 article.[22] Genovese argued that Cartwright was an influential physician whose theories aimed to naturalize and legitimize slavery in the U.S. South, whereas Haller proposed that Cartwright should be regarded as a controversial figure in the American medical profession, since he theorized on the basis of racial differences and enslaved people's mental and physical inferiority in comparison to those of Whites. Similarly, Stowe argued that Cartwright's theories on black bodies were founded upon preconceptions relating to slavery. Kenny showed how Cartwright and other southern physicians who studied black bodies in the 1840s and 1850s developed theories about enslaved people in an effort to modernize and revitalize the southern medical profession. Finally, Willoughby showed that while Cartwright's ideas circulated in southern political circles, they also had a broader impact on the northern medical profession and internationally. Willoughby therefore focused on Cartwright's impact on the more mainstream American medical profession, which is an aspect of Cartwright's life that has been overlooked in the historiography. While these scholars have tackled the circulation of Cartwright's ideas, his biography, and the content of his academic writings, few contributions have highlighted how Cartwright's theorizations of diseases such as drapetomania and dysaesthesia aethiopica not only helped popularize the theorization of black diseases within the American medical profession but also opened up new directions for the psychologizing of black behaviors in relation to stolen labor.

Cartwright was a successful doctor whose expertise was recognized by his peers in the South as well as in the North, which was not often the case for southern physicians. One of his articles received an award from the Medical Committee of Harvard University in 1826, and the *Boston Medical and Surgical Journal* (August 22, 1849) lauded his pamphlet entitled *Pathology and Treatment of Cholera,* saying that "such is the reputation of Dr. Cartwright for both professional skill and learning, that this publication is unquestionably exerting a commanding and sanitary influence in the region of the country for which it was prepared."[23] Cartwright was elected an honorary member of the Deinologian Society in 1833, one of the most active religious organizations in the South and a favorite of university professors, and also was elected to the Medical Society of the State of Virginia in 1843.[24] Throughout his medical career, Cartwright was known "as an able writer and medical philosopher, . . . extensively known throughout the South," who devoted his life to the understanding of southern ills, which were framed as "particular diseases."[25]

In addition, Cartwright was a steadfast advocate for the development of sectionalist medicine. In 1848, he pushed for the founding of southern medical societies, which would later be responsible for overseeing the dissemination of scientific productions from southern physicians and enslavers.[26] During his stay in Louisiana, Cartwright was named chairman of the Committee of the Medical Association of Louisiana to Report on Diseases of the Negro. Although he is sometimes described as having become "Professor of Diseases of the Negro," it is most likely that Cartwright did not have a tenured position at the Medical College of Louisiana (also known as the Medical Department of the University of Louisiana), since he was never listed as part of the medical faculty.[27]

One can explain the new theorization of the madness affecting black people by southern physicians such as Cartwright in the light of this issue of professionalization. The southern medical world was meeting a major challenge at the time: the need for recognition of southern physicians vis-à-vis their northern counterparts and the promotion of southern institutions in charge of training the future local medical elite in the management of what were seen as "specific diseases" affecting the populations of the South. At the time, the majority of Blacks resided mainly in the antebellum South; therefore, studying the diseases specific to this population, which was by definition "southern," justified, for local doctors, the creation of specific medical institutions in the South. The new theorizations of madness among black populations, and of other diseases seen as peculiar to this population, thus participated in and pro-longed the process of empowering southern medicine in relation to northern institutions.

Cartwright himself was a strong advocate for the rise of distinct southern medical institutions and expertise in the early 1850s. While studies of black be-havior were absent from medical journals in the North, Cartwright published an article in 1851 entitled "Report on the Diseases and Physical Peculiarities of the Negro Race" at the request of the State Medical Society, which had asked him to present his research at their annual symposium on March 12, 1851. In this article, Cartwright expressed his distress about the fact that the southern schools had not set up a single course on "black-specific disease education." To Cartwright, "no medical school was ever established near them [black people] until a few years ago; hence, their diseases and physical peculiarities are almost unknown to the learned."

Cartwright expressed regret that the few southern schools that had been founded in the late 1840s "should be content to linger behind those of the North" in terms of results and the number of students applying for admission, even though they had the opportunity to include in their school curricula in-formation about the 3 million Blacks who "were not cared for by any school." Introducing these courses, he continued, would have, in due time, placed the southern schools in the lead by attracting southern students who had previ-ously chosen to study in the North. Such a modification of school curricula "would be sending Science into a new field of usefulness," explained Cart-wright, convinced that southern medicine, when practiced widely by south-ern white doctors, could produce useful knowledge about Blacks, especially for the benefit of enslavers.[28] Therefore, Cartwright did not hide his ambitions for the social uses of medical science as he sought to align southern regionalist medicine with the southern moral, political, and social antebellum order.

In 1853, a correspondent of the same medical journal, Dr. Grier, expressed the same disbelief at the lack in southern medical schools of courses focused on black anatomy.[29] Grier recommended the training of professional physicians who could specifically deal with black bodies in the South. According to him, black diseases symbolized a peculiarity that justified the opening of new and exclusive medical sectors in the South, which in turn could only reinforce the prestige of these new regional institutions. Grier predicted that the medical schools in the South would then be "immediately crowded by a host of eager students from all parts of the slave-holding territory," thus defending the advent of southern medicine and, by extension, the potential for political applications of these medical theories, which would contribute to the strengthening of the southern social, moral, and political order in place.[30]

All in all, the defense of southern medical professionalism articulated by Grier and Cartwright reinforced the emerging antebellum political and economic culture of "southern distinctiveness," which arose from the development of a highly entrepreneurial class of planter-businessmen, whose fortunes were built on slavery, in the long nineteenth century.[31] Grier and Cartwright were both contemporaneous with the rise of the Democratic Party, which, since the 1840s, had become singularly devoted to promoting the defense and expansion of slavery and thus contributed to shaping a distinct political culture in the South, where Democrats had overwhelming support. For example, southern Democrats implemented specific legislative strategies on a federal scale, such as their push for the 1836–1844 gag rule, an effort to protect the interests of enslavers in Congress by postponing action on all petitions advocating against slavery, without hearing those petitions.[32] The Missouri Compromise of 1820 also reflected the long history of southern Democrats' obsession with the perceived abolitionist threat to their "way of life."[33]

The efforts of Cartwright and Grier to push for the development of distinct southern medical norms and subjects of study therefore paralleled broader southern political strategies surrounding slavery. Furthermore, the example of the medical trajectories of Grier and of Cartwright, one of the pioneers of the theory of madness affecting black populations, is evidence that there was indeed a link between the political and medical spheres.

Although Cartwright's political ideology was put under scrutiny, especially in the "burgeoning American print media," his close connection with the southern political elite has seldom been highlighted in previous works.[34] A fervent anti-abolitionist, Cartwright corresponded with Henry Clay, a senator and elected representative in Kentucky and the author of the Compromise of 1850. Clay, who earned the nickname "The Great Pacificator" after resolving the dispute between the free states and the slave states, wrote to Cartwright in 1844, six years before the passage of the compromise. Clay confided to Cartwright that he had "strong hopes that the spread of abolitionism may be greatly abated, if not extinguished in the North."[35]

In 1849, while debates between abolitionists and anti-abolitionists raged, Cartwright also entered into correspondence with Jefferson Davis. Cartwright was Jefferson Davis's personal physician and often provided him with medical advice.[36] In a letter written on June 10, 1849, Jefferson Davis expressed his disgust at seeing that in this "evil hour . . . some of the most distinguished of Southern Statesmen admitted that slavery was an evil." Davis could still count on his doctor and friend Cartwright to pay close attention to his political views: "To that, my doctor and friend, I do not believe it is a mistaken policy or a misguided humanity or an eager patriotism which conduits this crusade against our slave institution, but the strife for political dominion."[37]

Cartwright was also known to John A. Quitman, governor of Mississippi. Quitman sent a letter to Cartwright on October 2, 1850, in response to Cartwright's September 9 missive, which Quitman called "patriotic and philosophical." The governor sought to inform Cartwright of the latest news in Mississippi, which had been "the foremost in the protection of the rights of the South." Closely acquainted with Cartwright's ideas, Quitman congratulated himself for receiving Cartwright's "warm approbation of my course in attempting to uphold the noble position which our good state has taken in this slavery controversy." A convinced anti-abolitionist, Quitman sought during his term to advance the southern cause and lamented "attempts by deserters from the interests of the South to stifle truth, justice, patriotism and reason, by loud cheering, by firing of cannon and ringing of bells," which "will not do for a thinking and reflective people."[38]

"I trust we will yet show the Northern and Southern conspirators, that we have not to know the difference between a loaf of bread and a slave, or a fish and a serpent," Quitman explained in the same letter, acting as the spokesperson of enslavers who did not consider enslaved people to be anything but material goods. "With the exception of the merchants, hawkers, millionaires and their servile dependents, the people are opposed to submission," Quitman argued, assuring Cartwright that "this state will not quietly submit." Quitman could therefore rely on Cartwright to lend a sympathetic ear to his political views, since both men shared the same anti-emancipation ethos in the 1850s. Cartwright's theories quickly rallied new followers, who in turn imagined political applications of the medical theories published by the Louisiana physician. In August 1853, G. W. Marshall, a physician writing from Vicksburg, Mississippi, sent Cartwright a letter after reading his articles on the effects of alcoholism on the so-called deviant behavior of Blacks. "I send you a thousand thanks for so noble a contribution to the cause of science and humanity. They evince a singularly attentive observation upon current men and events and display an amount of labor and care for which very few Southern Physicians are distinguished. . . . I hope during the fall or early in the winter to see the whole series—of four numbers—embracing the 'Negro' number with the rest—put in pamphlet for general circulation," explained Marshall to Cartwright, enthusiastic about reading Cartwright's new scientific productions and seeing them widely circulated in the South.[39]

The exchange continued, and one year after this first letter, Marshall wrote to Cartwright to congratulate him for his most recent publication, telling him that he was "happy to inform you that on the main question I am heartily of your opinion. Slavery is right. It is of Divine appointment. It is neither an evil or a wrong. It is a blessing, rightly used to the white man; it is salvation and paradise to the Negro. And I hope the day is not far off when every Southerner who had any doubts or scruples on that subject will come to a sounder conviction and a better understanding of this momentous question."

Medical theories about black bodies and behaviors would be seen by Marshall as a political and ideological vector that could solidify the antebellum political order: "We must raise up Southern Teachers—we must print and publish our books and maintain the ancient renown and dignity of the South whose heads and hearts and harps and pens have molded the world."[40] This second letter shows that a real plan of action was organized by the southern doctors: the publication of southern medical theories and their distribution to help reaffirm southern sectionalist political power.

Following the advice of his friend Dr. Marshall, Cartwright undertook to better disseminate his theories on black bodies and, more particularly, on blackness and madness. On November 30, 1857, Cartwright delivered a landmark lecture to the New Orleans Academy of Sciences. The title of this conference was unequivocally racialist ("Ethnology of the Negro or Prognathous

Race"), and it was an attempt to draw up an inventory of the "different types of mankind." Cartwright divided mankind into three groups in the manner of Gobineau, who is cited in his paper. "The Indo-Europeans, the Mongolians and the Prognathous Race" all were depicted with fixed physical characteristics that were not modeled by the social environment or the climate in which they lived.

It is useful to observe here that Cartwright does not make any distinction between "Africans" and "slaves" in the United States; for him, they represent one and the same population, from which one can clearly deduce that he rejected outright any theories that took the environment into account. Cartwright would introduce the idea that Blacks belonged to the group he called the "prognathous race of mankind," which he defined as having inferior intellectual and moral characteristics in comparison to Indo-Europeans. "There is no office which the negro or mulatto covets more than that of being a body servant to a real gentleman. There is no office which gives him such a high opinion of himself, and it is utterly impossible for him to attach the idea of degredation [sic] to it. Those identical offices, which the white man instinctively abhors, are the most greedily sought for by negroes and mulattoes, whether slave or free, in preference to all other employments," Cartwright lectured the audience, insisting on the natural inferiority of the race. For Cartwright, enslaved people possessed an "innate love to act as body-servant or lacquey." Without this work of servitude, "his muscles not being exercised, the respiration is imperfect and the blood is imperfectly vitalized."

"Torpidity of body and hebetude of mind are the effects thereof, which disappear under bodily labor, because that expands the lungs, virilizes the blood and wakes him up to a sense of pleasure and happiness," Cartwright argued, trying to describe the mental and bodily changes that affected the constitution of the quintessential "black individual" when idle and not controlled by Whites. This first attempt at medicalizing and naturalizing the southern social order, however, seemed to focus wholly on the conditions of domestic servants, who were higher in the social hierarchy of the plantation, rather than addressing the case of field slaves.

In the second half of his lecture, however, Cartwright described cases of behavioral disorders and brain diseases specific to all enslaved people, regardless of their tasks, namely drapetomania, dysaesthesia aethiopica, and cachexia africana (also known as "negro consumption"). Cartwright presented to his peers in the medical profession the first disease, drapetomania, explaining that it manifested itself when enslaved people fled the plantation on which they resided. This flight constituted for Cartwright a state of "mental alienation," since the docility of Blacks and their submission to Whites was thought of as natural or innate. For Cartwright, the only possible cure for drapetomania was a paternalistic attitude of the enslaver toward the enslaved, whose senses were troubled. "If treated kindly, well fed and clothed, with fuel enough to keep a small fire burning all night—separated into families, each family having their own house—not permitted to run about at night, or to visit their neighbors, or to receive visits, or to use intoxicating liquors, and not overworked or exposed too much to the weather, they are very easily governed—more so than any other people in the world." However, if the state of alienation was ascertained, Cartwright recommended that those claiming property over recalcitrant enslaved people use corporal punishment "until they fall into that submissive state which it was intended for them to occupy in all after time, when their progenitor received the name of Canaan."

Cartwright also presented to his southern peers two new pathologies that were the cause of deviant behavior in black individuals: cachexia africana and dysaesthesia aethiopica, characterized by "hebetude of mind and insensibility of the body," which manifested itself when Whites gave too much work to the enslaved. "The empire of the white man's will over the prognathous race is not absolute, however. It cannot force exercise beyond a certain speed; neither the will nor physical force can drive negroes, for a number of days in succession, beyond a very moderate daily labor—about one-third less than what the white man voluntarily imposes on himself," Cartwright enunciated, thus always negatively comparing the physical and mental strength of the black man to that of the white man.

For Cartwright, these two mental deviations were evidence that Blacks could naturally attain a certain state of physical resistance, which turned out to be "an ample protection against the abuses of arbitrary power," and which justified, at the same time, their enslavement. Whereas "a white man, like a blooded horse, can be worked to death," Blacks, according to Cartwright, benefited from this instinctive resistance, which made them aware of when to stop working and thus preserve themselves for the tasks to come.[41]

Cartwright's published theories on insanity, labor, and racial preoccupations were also informed by the southern political economy and by the broader conversations about slavery that took place in the United States at the time. Cartwright's writings were published at a time marked by growth in the enslaved population of the Lower South. As historian Steve Deyle reveals, "between 1820 and 1860, at least 875,000 American slaves were forcibly removed from the Upper South to the Lower South."[42] The enslaved population grew rapidly between the 1830s and the 1850s. The 1830 U.S. census enumerated 2,009,043 enslaved people, whereas the 1850 census enumerated 3,204,313 enslaved people, a drastic increase of 37.3 percent.[43]

In fact, many new fortunes tied to slavery had been generated overnight in Cotton Kingdom states such as South Carolina. The Indian Removal Act of 1830 had paved the way for one of the largest and richest slave societies in history by allowing slavery to spread down into the Southwest, into Mississippi and Alabama, to cross the Mississippi River into Louisiana, and by the 1840s, to pour into Texas.[44] In this context of economic growth, white elite social circles in the South feared any unpredictability in the behavior of the enslaved. These elites were intimately concerned with the promotion and defense of slavery, since their source of income depended upon it. Fugitives from slavery were seen by enslavers as potential threats to the very institution of slavery and the moral order of the South.

It therefore comes as no surprise that Samuel Cartwright's theorization of drapetomania—a pathology he diagnosed with respect to fugitives from slavery—emerged in this specific context in the late 1850s. Drapetomania was theorized in the context of the Compromise of 1850, which comprised five laws that dealt with the issue of slavery and territorial expansion. Drafted to ease the increasing sectionalist tensions between the northern and southern states, the Compromise of 1850 guaranteed that California would enter the Union as a free state and that the slave trade would end in the District of Columbia, while promising that popular sovereignty would decide the question of slavery in the Utah and New Mexico territories. Furthermore, the compromise amended the Fugitive Slave Act, requiring northerners, after 1850, to help capture self-liberated individuals.[45] The act in its 1850 form gained much support from southern white elites because it drastically expanded their influence over northern states and promoted further control of the enslaved population. Cartwright's theorization of drapetomania can therefore be seen as an extension of the Fugitive Slave Act of 1850 to the medical sphere, as he proposed to pathologize self-emancipated individuals in a bid to restore the social and moral order reigning over southern plantations.

Cartwright's theories, which medicalized the black body, promulgate two stereotypes about blackness and labor that at first glance seem to contradict each other but which complement each other: labor is considered the innate activity that defines black experience, yet Blacks also are believed to demonstrate laziness as laborers. Interestingly, Cartwright's conflicting arguments complete the medical theories that had been championed in the early nineteenth century by Mississippi physician John Wesley Monette, who theorized black bodies as being idle, passive, and not virtuously hardworking.[46]

The two arguments, though completely opposite, could coexist. As historian Eugene Genovese contends, stereotypes about the laziness of Blacks and the theories about the laborious nature of enslaved people were commonplace in the eighteenth and nineteenth centuries. Whites often lamented the laziness of Blacks, as did enslaver Landon Carter, who, in Virginia in the eighteenth century, explained that he never saw "a short crop made so even by accident, ever managed either in time or really well."[47] Similarly, social critic Frederick Law Olmsted, visiting the South in the 1860s, observed that "slavery engendered deleterious, inefficient and slow work habits," pointing out that the enslaved were particularly slow to complete their tasks in comparison to northern workers.[48] These two arguments formed two sides of the same coin; they were the logical consequence of the latent paternalism that marked the relations between enslaved people and the enslavers in the antebellum South. The two arguments—that enslaved people are naturally lazy and that they are naturally inclined to work—complemented each other, as both defined Blacks as inherently inferior to Whites in all domains, according to different social contexts.

While theories about the mental abilities of Blacks were being developed and consolidated in the middle of the nineteenth century, especially in the writings of Samuel Cartwright, these theorizations of madness among black populations must be distinguished from the day-to-day practices of physicians when they treated black bodies on the plantations. Although the categories employed by Cartwright reveal how southern physicians politicized science to serve sectional interests, they were not made use of in the field. As historians Peter McCandless, Todd Savitt, Marli F. Weiner, and Mazie Hough have shown, mentally ill Blacks were not admitted to asylums and hospitals in large numbers prior to the 1850s.[49] In addition, drapetomania, dysaesthesia aethiopica, and cachexia africana are not mentioned in any institutional medical classifications.

In order to resolve this discrepancy between theory and practice, one can adopt the hypothesis, proposed by historian Katherine Bankole-Medina, that encounters between white doctors and Blacks were only sporadic and that southern physicians mainly focused on three issues. First, they sought to recruit cohorts of Blacks to consolidate classifications aimed at proving the biological inferiority of Blacks to Whites, which resulted in the publication of articles in medical journals by authors such as Cartwright in the 1850s. Second, they made routine visits to plantations or farms for the practical management of laboring black bodies. Third, the physicians maintained close contact with Blacks for reasons of ease of access—to practice medical experiments on them or on their corpses.[50] In general, therefore, theories about the intellectual abilities of Blacks informed medical practice but found no ready application in the field.[51]

However, this lack of application of medical theories in actual treatments does not mean that they did not have an impact on the regulation of plantation practices, especially since enslavers often consulted physicians such as Cartwright for advice regarding the health and the lack of docility of their enslaved workers. In fact, Cartwright was one of the first physicians in the South to fuel a specific rhetoric about manual labor and submissiveness toward Whites as defining the natural state of mind of Blacks. In his article "Ethnology of the Negro or Prognathous Race," he stated that "the ethnology of the prognathous race does not stop at proving that subordination to the white race is its normal condition" and that, according to him, "it goes further, and proves that social and political equality is abnormal to it, whether educated or not." He went on to hypothesize that, in consequence, "neither negroes nor mulattoes know how to use power when given to them."[52]

The pathologization of the black body and black behaviors that Cartwright undertook here served the financial interests of the white landowner (assuring him that the innate, biological nature of enslaved people was indeed to work), all while ensuring the medicalization of any potential black resistance or insubordination toward white enslavers, in order to anticipate any rebellions on the southern plantations. Slave rebellions in the 1840s and 1850s were a source of anxiety for white populations in southern states such as Louisiana, where enslavers would often recall the memory of the local slave insurrections of 1811.[53] Furthermore, slave rebellions were common in the 1850s, especially after the 1856 waves of slave rebellions in Missouri, Arkansas, and northern Louisiana.

The insurrections in Louisiana started as serious plots against enslavers in the parishes of St. Martin, Assumption, and St. Mary, not far from New Orleans, where Cartwright had his medical office.[54]

Relying on his reputation as one of the foremost black disease experts in Louisiana and the United States, Cartwright was able to position himself as a political expert, spreading his medical authority well beyond his medical prerogatives. All in all, Cartwright's theories, while being deeply linked to the southern political order, aimed to transform black bodies into laborious masses, with the aim of extracting enslaved people's physical forces and stealing their labor to advance the productivity of the plantation system. By doing so, Cartwright put forth theories linking race to madness and forced labor, which would have a long-lasting impact on post–Civil War protopsychiatric theories about black bodies. Furthermore, Cartwright's ongoing conversations with Louisiania physicians such as G. W. Marshall and S. L. Grier, and with statesmen such as Jefferson Davis and John A. Quitman, further highlight that his theories and political beliefs operated within a network of influence, thus helping his theories to circulate in the local medical profession.

Before the publication of Cartwright's theories, enslaved people were rarely declared insane in the southern states, where most of the black population was concentrated. As historian Peter McCandless has shown, such diagnoses had been made more frequently (though still only sporadically) when the southern colonies were still under British rule, before the Declaration of Independence. However, despite the use of this classification, enslaved people would not often get treatments for insanity on the plantations or in state institutions. For example, Kate, an enslaved woman in South Carolina, was put in prison under the authority of Craven County after being suspected of murdering a black child in 1745 and was classified as being "out of her senses." She remained in jail without receiving any care, because South Carolina had not established any provision for enslaved people suffering from madness, and her owner, Robert Fullwood, was far too poor to pay the fees for her release.[55] This case led to the creation of a 1745 South Carolina law that ruled that any enslaved person in a similar case would be placed in detention without the possibility of bail, thus resolving the question of whether he or she would be placed in a state institution, should the enslaver be unable to contribute financially to his or her commitment to an asylum.[56] The measures taken by the state of South Carolina would therefore provide a solution regarding the isolation of an enslaved individual deemed to be insane and potentially dangerous, by removing them from the plantation; however, it did not provide any treatment or possibility of transformation for the diseased individual.

The concept of madness affecting black populations therefore existed, but it was not tied to any specific theorization. The enslaved individual was put away without any specific mention of mental care. On the other hand, an enslaved person qualified as "out of their senses" was judged on the basis of what was considered their usual behavior. For example, the physicians viewed work to be an expression of "natural" behavior, and a refusal to work would therefore be the mere expression of a passing folly, something on the order of a child misbehaving or not knowing what is good for them. Their condition was not judged in terms of pathologies, since no proper medical treatment was ever envisioned or provided before the 1850s.

Since enslaved people were considered property and suffered a situation that sociologist Orlando Patterson describes as "social death," enslavers ultimately saw little reason to count them as mentally ill or to summon a medical expert.[57] As a result, enslaved people often developed their own alternative medicine to care for each other on the plantations, especially in the case of physical injuries related to work, or exhaustion.[58] In some cases, enslaved people classified by overseers or medical officers as insane continued, to a certain extent, to perform activities for the benefit of enslavers. Enslaved women thus classified, for instance, worked as nurses to ensure the breast-feeding of young white children, their mental health not being considered in the assignment of this task by the enslavers.[59]

Moreover, it was not in the interest of enslavers to declare enslaved people to be mentally ill, as it would drastically reduce their monetary value in the case of sale. Examination of the bills of trade for the public sales of the enslaved in Louisiana makes it readily apparent that enslaved people classified as lunatic were much cheaper than others on sales lists and therefore represented a financial loss for their owner; hence the need to avoid this classification to maximize sales gains.[60] This fact has often been overlooked in the historiography. Enslavers also marked "sound and healthy" on coupons they signed to assure their buyers that the enslaved individual in question did not present any particular disorder. In the absence of this mention, the enslaved person could be returned to his master of origin and the notarial act annulled. In New Orleans on May 13, 1847, for example, Edouard Rieffel sold to Joseph Bruneau an enslaved man named George, aged about twenty-nine years, for the sum of $550; however, a few months later, George was sent back to Rieffel and the sale was canceled because he was not considered fit for work by Bruneau, who declared that he was "insane" (*fou,* in the French original).[61]

Furthermore, each day of rest signified a financial loss, and if enslavers granted a period of rest to an enslaved worker, they feared it would encourage further requests, and perhaps even rebellion. Convalescence was thus rarely prescribed or was nonexistent for mental illnesses. In a report written in the 1860s detailing the history of care provided in Louisiana, Dr. Delery wrote that enslaved people "do become insane as well as other persons, and in the same proportion," and that their enslavers "are not prompted by the ordinary instincts of humanity, or disregarding their own interest, they are not willing to incur the expense of $150 per annum, in having them provided with the means most likely to restore them to a state of sanity."[62]

For economic reasons, then, madness among black populations was rarely treated. The planters did not want to take enslaved people to the hospital because it represented a significant cost. Enslaved people, whether men or women, represented only a malleable work force for them. The enslaved person could, however, be treated for physical ailments, if it enabled him to be put back on his feet so he could resume his labor. Some of the enslaved were sent to centers like the Touro Infirmary for injuries, while doctors were sometimes called to plantations to treat injured or contagious patients.[63]

Although institutionalization for enslaved people affected by mental disorders was rare, some in the 1840s were treated for madness in institutions such as the Eastern Lunatic Asylum in Williamsburg. Built in 1773, the Eastern Lunatic Asylum was the first public asylum in Virginia, and indeed was one of the first asylums in the United States.[64] Enslaved people were institutionalized in the asylum in the early 1840s, when its director, John Minson Galt II, argued that his institution should accept Whites, free Blacks, and enslaved people, in contrast to the admission policies of the second Virginia facility, the Western State Lunatic Asylum, erected in Staunton in 1828, which treated only white patients.[65]

As historian Wendy Gonaver has shown, Galt's argument for the inclusion of enslaved people within the asylum's walls was instrumental in changing the asylum's demography. In response to Galt, the Virginia State Assembly, elected in March 1841, decided to formally facilitate the admission of free Blacks and enslaved people to the Eastern Lunatic Asylum, provided they remained in the minority, did not live near white patients, and the medical staff prevented "any disadvantage occurring to the white patients from the presence of the other race." The state assembly further argued that "$8,000 should be appropriated by the legislature, if [the physicians] wished to carry out promptly and efficiently the benevolent purpose which they have voluntarily formed."

The act stipulated that the costs incurred by enslaved people in the establishment should be paid by the enslaver or by whoever was responsible for them.[66] The enslavers were to pay the sum of $2.00 per week for each enslaved man taken in charge by the asylum and $1.50 per enslaved woman. Following the passage of the law, Galt signed an act, in 1841, stipulating that enslavers placing enslaved people into the asylum should provide payment "for board and clothes for the said patient at the rate of one dollar and fifty cents a week . . . and shall remove or pay the expenses of the removal or the said patient, whenever this is required by the Superintendent of the said asylum and shall also pay for one entire suit of clothes to be finished to the said patient on discharge." The financial conditions were different if a family member chose to commit to the same institution a patient who was not enslaved: they should pay "board for the said patient, at the rate of four dollars a week and all necessary expenses for clothing . . . and shall remove or pay the expenses of the removal of the said patient whenever this is required by the Superintendent of the said asylum."[67]

What is little known is that, for Galt, the real novelty of the law lay in the admission of enslaved people to the asylum in 1841, since they had never previously been officially accepted into such an institution. Writing a note in his records in 1841, Galt, who had just become the medical superintendent at the age of twenty-two, explained that his institution had always admitted free black patients because other asylums in Virginia, such as the Western Lunatic Asylum, refused to take them—a fact which has been overlooked in the recent historiography. Galt argued that his "institution has always taken insane free blacks; the laws respecting the admissions of white pauper lunatics, having been ever confined to apply to all free persons of whatever race they might be" and that "no difference has ever been made in this respect between applications coming from the one class of patients or from the other." Galt enthusiastically explained that "since March 6th 1841, no application, we may state, for the reception of a colored patient had been rejected," and that while "the Western Asylum refused to take colored patients, the Eastern Institution may be supposed to accommodate all the free blacks in Virginia who are suitable objects for such a charity." The real change was that "slaves have never enjoyed its benefits, doubtless from the fact that there was no legal permission for this." Galt further stated that he could perceive "no reason why insane slaves should not be permitted thus to obtain relief of their sad diseases."[68] According to him, free Blacks had always been welcomed in his institution before 1841, on the condition that they paid their medical treatments:

> Virginia having a free colored population larger than any other slave state save one, necessarily offers us a good example with reference to the subject of consideration, and any conclusion which we may arrive at must be considered as applicable also to the other states respecting the same social organization. The Eastern asylum is the recipient of all free colored persons deemed by the magistrates fit subjects for such a destination; no insane individual of this class has been rejected for several years past, by reason of the want of room and the laws at present entirely favour the admission of all such patients.[69]

Even though free Blacks were a small minority of the population in Virginia and other southern states, Galt offered recommendations and special provisions for the few of them suffering from mental afflictions, in order to welcome them in the institution he supervised.[70] He headed a committee that ruled in favor of the creation of separate wards for black patients, free or enslaved, in Virginia as early as 1844. This testifies to the longevity of such a debate, which began long before the creation of the nation's first asylum for black patients, the Central Lunatic Asylum, in Virginia, in 1869.[71] If Galt was not the medical superintendent who changed the modalities of internment of black patients at the Eastern Lunatic Asylum, he was the one who pushed for the cure and institutionalization of enslaved people.

The documents left by John Galt also shed light on the debates concerning racial diversity in his asylum in the 1840s. In his report to the Virginia assembly, Galt did not advocate the construction of a separate new institution for free or enslaved black people in the state.[72] Galt enumerated three main moral obstacles that, according to him, would undermine the success of such a segregated institution. First, the recruitment of a director for such an institution would be problematic, because the asylum would be small, with only a few patients to be in charge of, and so the salary paid to the director would be correspondingly low: "When we come to consider that according to what we have previously stated [the fact that there are fewer Blacks than Whites suffering from mental afflictions in the state of Virginia], such an institution must be small, and hence as an almost necessary consequence, the salary of a superintendent would be low."

Second, according to Galt, the public would take little interest in this institution for Blacks. Galt feared that "less interest would be taken by the public in asylums strictly established, for the colored race, than for those receiving both kinds of patients: and consequently, there would exist a greater liability to neglect, misrule and abuse than could occur under the opposite system, by reason of an interested and searching public opinion, and constant public observation of insanity." Therefore, Galt was concerned with how Black patients (whether free or enslaved) would be treated in a separate institution, arguing that any bad management on the asylum administrators' part would therefore go unchecked.

Third, for him, the number of free Blacks and enslaved people in Virginia who were classified as insane was hardly sufficient to justify the establishment of such a facility in 1844. To support his reasoning, Galt relied not on federal statistics but on the statistics of his institution, arguing that only twelve free black women and five free black men were residing in his institution, which indicated that the construction of an asylum dedicated to treating Blacks was not necessary for a population so restricted: "To show how little then a separate institution is desirable for these lunatics in the South, it is not necessary to go further into statistics, than simply to state that there are in the Eastern Asylum only twelve free colored females and five males." Galt explained that the cost of housing black patients in an asylum specifically open to them would in the long run require too much capital investment from the state of Virginia.

Later on, Galt would also cite the small number of lunatics present in the northern states, relying on the 1840 census returns about race and insanity to prove that, after all, the madness of the Blacks was not ultimately a problem that required the building of separate institutions in Virginia or in any other state of the Union. Using examples taken from New England institutions, Galt argued that investing in the construction of a separate asylum for black patients was not necessary, given the small number of Blacks suffering from insanity in the country: "In the Maine State Hospital, only one insane colored person was ever admitted as a patient, only one has been admitted into the New Hampshire asylum, and no application has ever been made to the Vermont asylum for a patient of this class." As we will see in chapter 2, these census returns were used in southern anti-abolitionist circles to naturalize the link between race and insanity and to argue that enslaved people were less affected by madness than free Blacks in the North because emancipation provoked episodes of insanity. Galt relied on these statistics to argue that "so few cases of insanity would occur amongst such limited numbers as these, that the question of separate asylums does not apply to them" and that "the number of insane free colored persons is too small to justify the expense of a separate asylum" in Virginia. Galt chose to comment upon New England institutions to expand his argument that separate institutions were not needed in Virginia, not because racial separation or segregation was a moral wrong but because of financial concerns.

Thus, Galt did not oppose having black patients in his institution; quite the contrary. In the rest of his report to the committee, Galt pointed out that black and white inmates should be cared for in a single institution, such as the Eastern Lunatic Asylum where he was the director. He also recommended that other southern states follow his model of racial diversity in asylums.

While formulating this opinion, which favored racial integration within a state institution, Galt was aware of the strong criticism that hung over his argument. First, he admitted that white and black inmates, by their newfound proximity, would be likely to befriend each another, which could "materially interfere with the comfort, the management and the cure of both white and colored patients." Second, the organization of a racially mixed asylum "might create in the public mind, on account of the general prejudice on the subject, an unfavorable impression against any asylum so constituted." Third, Galt conceded that employees would be mostly employed in the care of white patients, and that finding good employees devoted to the care of black patients could become a problem. According to Galt, white employees (such as nurses and physicians) would be tempted "in a greater degree to revenge the insulting expressions, demeanor and conduct of colored than of white patients."

These reservations, however, were put into perspective by Galt, and their importance minimized. According to him, black and white patients could feasibly cohabit in a single asylum. First, he argued, black and white inmates did not come into contact with each other inside his institution, and he pointed out that in the case of lunatics with forms of dementia, their illness made them forget their promiscuity, since "lunatics laboring under dementia take less notice, as a general rule, of their situation and companions than those affected with the other varieties of insanity." Galt concluded that "in case the colored insane were admitted amongst white patients," white lunatics would not necessarily interact with them, "provided it was not considered proper to locate them on the same or nearly the same footing as white patients." Second, Galt pointed out that the asylum space could very easily be organized to minimize contact between white and black patients because "the insane have generally little intercourse and conversation with their companions and are not inclined to take much notice of them."

"In the Eastern asylum of Virginia, no peculiar strictness is observed in [illegible] the white from the colored patients; nor under the arrangement adopted in this respect, is there the slightest difficulty in management, originating from the presence of the two races in the same asylum," explained Galt. He further argued that since "the male colored are few, being ordinarily only half the number of the females belonging to this class, . . . no special arrangement was adopted with respect to them." He added, "For very few of the male patients are in the wards but a short time during the day, so that except in rare instances, there is little or no necessary direct communication between the two classes." Clearly, Galt was eager to prove that racial mixing within the asylum's walls was not a constraint for the staff. Finally, Galt explained, white patients equated black patients with enslaved people who worked within the institution, thereby increasing the distance between these two categories of inmates: "The servants of the institution are all of them slaves, and the white patients are familiar of course with these, and generally look upon the colored patients pretty much in the same light as they do the servants."[73]

Among other things, Galt's argument in support of the racial integration of the southern institutions highlights the exceptional character of the admission of free and enslaved Blacks, who were not very numerous in his institution in the 1840s. This observation corroborates the data gathered by historian Peter McCandless, which indicates that the South Carolina Lunatic Asylum hosted enslaved people as patients as early as 1829 but that these patients only came episodically, their admission being poorly encouraged by the law.[74] As long as black patients were neither numerous nor in the majority in institutions, racial integration was tolerated during the antebellum period, throughout which the diagnosis of madness among black populations had still to be systematized.

However, it is important to note that Galt's regimen of treatment regarding race and madness was far from being widely followed or systematized; it constituted an exception in nineteenth-century medicine and was far from being the rule in the pre–Civil War era. Galt's reformist ideas also must be nuanced, given what has been previously said about him in the historiography. Though he was close to abolitionist movements and decided to support the internment of a minority of black patients within his asylum, this did not necessarily mean that his aim was to promote interracial institutions or interracial contact within the asylum.[75] Indeed, the last three quotes from Galt mentioned here show that Blacks were not admitted on an equal footing with white patients, and that black patients were tolerated as long as they remained "few" compared to Whites.

By 1861, forty-eight asylums had opened in the United States. One of them had been created by the federal government; twenty-seven others by the assemblies of twenty-one states in total. Five were funded and controlled by cities and counties in four states, and the remaining fifteen were private institutions.[76] In certain cases, and according to certain prerogatives, notably in the Virginia asylum, enslaved people were institutionalized in small numbers, but mostly after the 1840s.

We have seen here that madness was a pathology that was only gradually applied to Blacks over the nineteenth century. This highlights the shifting and sometimes conflicting nature of scientific theorizations. As French historians Christophe Prochasson and Anne Rasmussen point out, science has always been shaped by scientific controversies, which end up being "rhetorical and argumentative resources" and which allow "the laborious emergence of reason, which is the fruit of a dialectical work resulting from the confrontation of the arguments, from where the solution arises."[77] The theorizations around the madness of Blacks did not escape this rule; they were at the core of the political debate in which monogenists and polygenists, southerners and northerners, all confronted one another.

When theories about madness were perceived to be a legitimate field of expertise for southern doctors such as Samuel Cartwright, madness was gradually recognized as an eminently political disease, in that its successive theorizations reflected political and medical sectionalist issues. As an unintentional consequence of subverting Dorothea Dix's theory, madness would give Blacks a semblance of humanization; and in defiance of this, madness was for many years rejected as a diagnosis by white doctors, until it was theorized by southern physicians such as Cartwright in the 1840s, whose aim was to intervene in the political debates of the South and to build an autonomous southern field of medicine, independent from northern practices and institutions. Cartwright's plans were also concomitant with the southern political economy of the time, as Democrats sought to preserve the moral, social, economic, and political order of the antebellum South at all costs.

The invention of madness as a disorder affecting black populations also took place within the broader moral and political economy that structured the evolution of theories of alienation, the use of forced labor as moral treatment, and nineteenth-century care practices. The enslavers did not call upon doctors to treat the madness of enslaved people because they considered the cost too high. This partly explains the absence of any systematic pathologization of Blacks suffering from mental afflictions in the antebellum medical literature. And because they were not sent in significant numbers to the institutions of the country, the madness of Blacks was not construed as a genuine public concern.[78]

Chapter 2 will address the changes wrought when madness is presented as a public concern, which became the case after the publication of the 1840 census, which showed a steady increase in the number of Blacks suffering from madness in both the North and the South. The gradual dissemination of the interwoven medical arguments tying up race and madness, which would be put into practice in southern medical institutions in the post–Civil War era, will be discussed in this and subsequent chapters.

2

THE STRANGE CAREER
OF THE 1840 CENSUS STATISTICS

It was the census that was insane, and not the colored people.

—REV. JAMES FREEMAN CLARKE, "Condition of the Free Colored People
of the United States," *Christian Examiner* (1859)

T he 1840s were the theater of a compelling debate surrounding the state
of mind of free black individuals residing in the free states.[1] The 1840
census showed, for the first time in American history, a stark contrast
between numbers of black individuals who were classified as insane in the
North and in the South. In the free northern states, the 1840 census recorded
that one free black person in every 143 black inhabitants was insane, while in
the slave states, the ratio dropped down to only one in every 1,605 enslaved
people, which seemed to suggest that insanity affecting black individuals was
much more prevalent in territories where they were free.[2]

As soon as the 1840 census results started to circulate, northern and southern physicians alike noticed the stark contrast between the number of black
people listed as "insane" or "idiot" in the northern states and those listed as
such in the South. Reading the statistics in 1842, Edward Jarvis, a physician
originally from Massachusetts who was living in Kentucky, claimed enthusiastically that the census returns showed that "slavery has a wonderful influence
upon the development of moral faculties and the intellectual powers," given
the fact that black men and women seemed to be less prone to insanity in the
South than in the North.[3]

The census statistics from 1840 would inspire physicians for decades. In the
1880s and 1890s, J. F. Miller, the superintendent of the Eastern North Carolina

Insane Asylum in Goldsboro, North Carolina; T. O. Powell, superintendent of the Georgia Lunatic Asylum; W. F. Drewry, superintendent of the Central State Hospital at Petersburg, Virginia; E. D. Bondurant, assistant superintendent of the Alabama Insane Hospital; and T. J. Mitchell, superintendent of the Mississippi State Lunatic Asylum, all discussed the rates of insanity affecting Blacks throughout the South. All used successive census returns, starting with the 1840 census, combined with statistics from their local institutions, to put forward the hypothesis that formerly enslaved black people and their descendants had rapidly become "insane" as they were not able to handle their status as freedmen and freedwomen.[4]

Although the production of these political statistics in the 1840s has been discussed in groundbreaking book chapters and articles, little light has been cast either on the aftermath or on the revival of the statistics of insanity affecting black individuals in the antebellum and postbellum eras. Most of the scholarship published about these census statistics on insanity was published by historians of the U.S. census, who focused on the production of data and the statistical errors made by official census representatives instead of on the circulation of these statistics within broad medical, political, and media circles over the decades that followed their publication. For example, the first historian to look at the 1840 census, Albert Deutsch, published an article in 1944 in which he claimed that the statistics on insanity affecting Blacks were purposefully produced and manipulated for use in proslavery arguments. Historian Leon Litwack also briefly referenced the 1840 census statistics in an effort to show how the statistics had fostered vivid debates in Congress between 1842 and 1845. Historian of science Theodore Porter chose to discuss the 1840 census statistics on insanity to show how they paved the way for a new era of social statistics in the country.[5]

In 1999, Margo Anderson and Stephen E. Fienberg included several pages on the 1840 census and on statistics of insanity affecting Blacks, mainly to summarize the debates on census accuracy, in a book that explored the origins and history of the census.[6] More recently, historians Patricia Cline Cohen and Paul Schor have examined the hypothesis that data had been intentionally manipulated in the 1840 census. Their findings show instead that the 1840 census statistics were riddled with successive errors. For a start, William A. Weaver, in charge of the census of 1840, noted that there had been irregularities but pleaded ignorance, explaining that he had not had time to look at the figures before they were published. Indeed, John Quincy Adams had lobbied in the summer of 1841 to obtain census results faster than initially planned, and this haste is one of the potential causes of the large number of errors in the 1840 census, as the results had not yet been "digested." Following Cohen's and Schor's arguments, it is unlikely that the statistical results were deliberate manipulations or were engineered for propaganda purposes; the errors were simply the result of incompetence, because Weaver had surrounded himself with a poorly trained team to handle the production of census statistics and was himself a novice.[7]

While taking into consideration these successive and important research findings, this chapter focuses on the politicization of medical theories on insanity affecting black individuals, from the 1840s to the 1890s, following the publication of the 1840 census. I will not examine how these numbers were produced, as this has been the topic of many books and articles published in the field of the history of science.[8] Rather, through the examination of various and sometimes contradictory arguments, I aim to show how the census became an institution and a battlefield that pushed physicians and political commentators to shape various political interpretations of insanity, in both the antebellum and postbellum eras, until the 1890s. Making use of several disciplines—the history of science, history of medicine, and history of race relations in the Old South and the New South—this chapter offers an analysis of the political economy of insanity in relation to sectionalism. I will examine how southern physicians used their scientific legitimacy and authority as public figures to condemn black people's freedom in the North before 1865, and then the civil rights gained by newly freed individuals during and after Reconstruction in the South.

The 1840 census returns on insanity first became the object of public scrutiny with the publication of an article on September 21, 1842, by Edward Jarvis in the *Boston Medical and Surgical Journal,* one of the first and most prestigious medical journals founded in the United States.[9] Born in Massachusetts, Jarvis was a physician who had graduated from Harvard in 1826. After serving as an apprentice at the office of a local physician, Jarvis trained at the Harvard Medical School, where he received his degree in 1830. He was living in Louisville, Kentucky, in 1842 when he laid hands on the first edition of the 1840 census returns published by Blair and Rives.[10] Respected in his field, Jarvis was an elected member of the American Statistical Association, and his work as a physician was often cited by his peers in the pages of the oldest and most prestigious journals of medicine, including the *Philadelphia Medical Journal*. Intrigued by the census figures on madness, Jarvis immediately decided to write on the causes of the madness of Whites and Blacks, using the newly published raw census data.

Jarvis began his article with a close examination of some errors that he had found in the 1840 census tables. His article included a table listing the returns from the northern and southern states, and he pointed out that federal marshals sent to Massachusetts to collect the data had greatly underestimated the number of individuals classified as insane, when compared to the local statistics collected by the directors of the asylums. According to Jarvis, this was due to the fact that the marshals "must obtain all their knowledge second hand; and as many look at insanity as stigma on the family, even disgraceful, they are often unwilling to report to a stranger the fact that one in their household is insane, or an idiot." For Jarvis, the stigma of madness distorted the survey, and he believed that local administrators or overseers of asylums, for example, were in a better position to report the numbers than the U.S. marshals or their assistants, who had no connection to the local population.

Therefore, the rationalization of the results, as undertaken by Jarvis, focused on the causes of underreporting in the field and, in particular, the weight of the different social interactions in the shaping of statistics. Despite the demonstration of these early mistakes and inconsistencies, Jarvis did not disapprove of the 1840 census. Instead, he announced that it was a document "equally true in all its parts," since, according to him, the errors balanced themselves out. This fact is not often reported in the secondary literature that deals with this material. Jarvis's purpose was more to defend the honor and the legitimacy of the document than to fundamentally question or undermine it.

However, in that same article, Jarvis noted a quite astonishing statistical dynamic: according to him, the census showed "a vast difference between the condition of the colored men in the free states and that in the slave states." Noting that there was a "ten-fold proportion of colored insane in the free, above that in the slave states," Jarvis argued that the large numbers of lunatics in the population proved that slavery removed enslaved people from the danger of more mental excitement and daily worries than their minds (judged too little inclined to complexity) could handle: "Slavery has a wonderful influence upon the development of moral faculties and the intellectual powers; and refusing man many of the hopes and responsibilities which the free, self-thinking and self-acting enjoy and sustain, of course it saves him from some of the liabilities and dangers of active self-direction." Jarvis further argued that "so far as this goes, it proves the common notion that in the highest state of civilization and mental activity there is the greatest danger of mental derangement; for here, where there is the greatest mental torpor, we find the least insanity," making a link between blackness and a "lack of civilization," which supposedly would explain why the sanity of enslaved people in the South was preserved. Jarvis concluded that since "there are many other considerations to be taken into the account, . . . the whole subject of the effect of slavery, in all its bearings, upon mental health, is worth an extensive and thorough investigation, which we have not space here to pursue," thus pushing for more investigations into the matter.

Interestingly, Jarvis here considered a lack of "civilization" to be preventative against insanity. According to him, slavery, the equivalent of a lack of civilization, allowed black individuals to remain in a mental state that was not dangerous to themselves or to others. This argument echoed one of the most common opinions already circulating in the medical field of the time about insanity and civilization. In the light of these arguments, it appears clear that Jarvis was the first to accept the results of the 1840 census without paying attention to potential inconsistencies in the census tables. Having no time himself to dwell on this new cause of insanity, Jarvis invited doctors to conduct research on the issue.[11]

The editors of the *Southern Literary Messenger*, a journal that printed poetry, historical notes, and nonfiction, quickly followed up on Jarvis's proposition. In June 1843, the journal published "Reflections on the Census of 1840," which strongly supported the hypothesis that these statistics demonstrated a natural incapacity on the part of Blacks to adapt to freedom. The article developed a lengthy discussion of the "dark shades" in the American picture as the "census exhibits a startling amount of insanity among our people." Surprised by the census figures, the author undertook to rationalize them by stating that the spread of madness among black individuals seemed to correspond to the number of years of emancipation, thus following Jarvis's line of argument. "It is a remarkable fact, that where slavery had been longest extinguished, the condition of the colored race is worse." The author took the example of the numbers in "Massachusetts and Maine," where slavery "has been extinguished more than half a century," as well as in New Hampshire and Vermont, where "there have not been more than eight slaves at any time, within the last forty years," to show that "throughout this region the amount of insane in the colored class is 1 in 34," which therefore proved that, according to him, freedom brought mental ills to formerly enslaved people in proportion to the number of years that they had been freed.[12]

Further on in the text, the author described madness affecting black populations as a threat to public order, invoking the image of bloodthirsty and savage hordes rising in the country, and the author did not hesitate to evoke the uprisings of enslaved people against the British in Jamaica to fuel the *Messenger's* dystopian vision. The *Southern Literary Messenger* article remains the first to use the viciousness and profligacy argument to expose how madness affecting black individuals diverges "naturally" from madness affecting Whites. The author again relied on statistics, this time produced by the penitentiary system of Pennsylvania, concerning "vicious" free black individuals, "the increase of which and the evils thereof, are obvious to all." The author described the black population of Pennsylvania as "profligate," suffering from idleness, compared to those of Virginia, a slave state of the Old South, who were proportionately much less numerous in the state's penitentiary system. The *Southern Literary Messenger* article also instrumentalized the insanity of mulattoes to further the argument that interracial relationships were unnatural, since "those of mixed blood are more liable to insanity than the pure Africans," and would lead to "the ruin of the nation."

Finally, in the last part of the article, the author made a dozen propositions summarizing his arguments. Madness, he stated, derives from "vicious habits and uncontrolled passions," and not from "the effect of climate," since "the black man enjoys as good health, as far as climate is concerned, as the white, on every part of this continent." The principle of temporality was also discussed, as "the vices of the free blacks have increased in proportion to the time that has elapsed since their emancipation," while the need to forbid intermarriages was formulated as follows: "Intermarriage between the white and black races is unnatural, contrary to the order and design of Providence, and fatal to posterity, in inducing disease and premature death." In summary, the author argued that "general emancipation would be attended with the most severe consequences to the country where it would take place, and eventually prove fatal to the emancipated race."[13]

The piece from the *Southern Literary Messenger* was circulated in southern circles. The same month it was published, it was quoted in the *Daily National Intelligencer* in Washington, DC, in an article titled "Curious Statistical Facts."[14] These statistics could have remained hidden in a set of obscure, forgotten publications, but events took another turn as proslavery apologists eagerly seized upon the numbers as scientific confirmation that black people had a natural propensity to enslavement. Former vice president John C. Calhoun, a notorious supporter of slavery and himself an enslaver, enthusiastically jumped upon the opportunity offered by the 1840 census figures to provide scientific proof of the natural inferiority of the "black man." Writing in 1844 to Richard Pakenham, the British ambassador to the United States, Calhoun claimed that the census results showed that freedmen "have been invariably sunk into vice and pauperism, accompanied by the bodily and mental inflictions incident thereto—deafness, blindness, insanity and idiocy—to a degree without example."[15] Calling the census an "authentic document," Calhoun argued that since Blacks had lived in slave states and had submitted to the "ancient relation," "they have improved greatly in every respect—in number, comfort, intelligence, and morals." To Calhoun, the longer slavery had been abolished, the worse the mental condition of Blacks had become, thus forging direct causal links between temporality, freedom, and madness.

Calhoun's position regarding the statistics was no surprise, considering his pivotal role in South Carolina's 1832 secession movement. A defender of slavery and of white supremacy, Calhoun took part in the nullification crisis of 1828–1833, which was a confrontation between the state of South Carolina and the federal government over South Carolina's attempt to declare null and void the 1828 and 1832 federal tariffs within the state. Calhoun's labored concerns about states' rights during the crisis show his militancy in defending southern interests, in the context of widespread criticism of slavery in the North.[16]

Calhoun's defense of the argument that freedom created mental illness for Blacks was not an isolated phenomenon in the 1840s. Many white southern Democratic leaders were increasingly becoming worried that the phenomenal wealth and political power the Deep South had amassed in such a short time would disappear if northerners successfully challenged the legality of slavery. White southerners turned to naturalists, physicians, and preachers who claimed to be experts about black behaviors and black bodies in order to legitimize their claims that enslaved people were naturally fitted for unsophisticated tasks and manual labor.[17] In the nineteenth century, before the Civil War, as historian Stephen R. Haynes has noted, proslavery apologists often would cite passages from the book of Genesis, such as the cursing of Ham (or Canaan) in Genesis 9, to justify slavery.[18]

Similarly, phrenology, which was pioneered by Viennese naturalist Franz Joseph Gall, was used in scientific circles to demonstrate the inferiority of non-white races. Kentucky-born physician Charles Caldwell used phrenology to attempt to prove that African peoples were naturally suited for manual labor, and therefore for slavery, while physiologist Samuel G. Morton helped justify Andrew Jackson's forced displacement of Native Americans from their land in the 1830s by arguing that the mental capacities of Indigenous peoples were not aligned with the processes of industrialization and progress.[19] In 1854, southern physicians Josiah C. Nott and George R. Gliddon published *Types of Mankind*, which was heavily influenced by Morton's writings, in an effort to attempt to prove that inferior races were more closely linked to animals.[20] Consequently, the debates over the soundness of free and enslaved black individuals bore the mark of political urgency, as white southerners became increasingly desperate in the 1850s to embrace any proof that slavery was not only a way of life but also a political necessity.

Calhoun had long given his vocal support to the belief that races could be distinguished by their intellectual and physical characteristics. In his speech on the reception of abolition petitions in the District of Columbia in 1837, he stated that the attack of the abolitionists on the slaveholding institution was a "systematic design of rendering [the South] hateful in the eyes of the world— with a view to a general crusade."[21] Well aware of the abolitionists' claims that slavery was inhumane, Calhoun nonetheless argued that the "peculiar institution of the South" should prevail because "the existing relation between the two races in the South, against which these blind fanatics are waging war, forms the most solid and durable foundation on which to rear free and stable political institutions." He justified this claim by saying that "the political condition of the slaveholding states has been so much more stable and quieter than that of the North." In a way, Calhoun's use of federally produced objective numbers allowed him to sustain his dystopian tale, which pictured a vulnerable white society directly threatened by the impetuosity and brutality of black freedom. Furthermore, Calhoun's comments on the 1840 census show a deliberate intention to politicize the medicalization of insanity affecting black individuals, in the context of rising tensions between the North and the South.

In the northern states and abroad, divergent voices emerged to condemn the proslavery use of these statistics. The statistics eventually crossed the Atlantic, and in 1843, a Spanish physician, Ramón de la Sagra, published an essay about the "worrisome numbers" on insanity affecting Blacks in the United States. De la Sagra was a botanist, economist, and anarchist essayist from Galicia who in 1845 founded the newspaper *El Porvenir,* which was later considered the world's first anarchist newspaper. He was close to Pierre-Joseph Proudhon and was interested in medicine, which he had studied before moving to France. Though he was respected in both Europe and the United States, his work on the 1840 census remains unknown to historians to this day, even though the tenor of his argument is so very different from that of his American counterparts. He published in French; it was not uncommon to see the first journals of Francophone medicine and psychiatry, such as the *Archives générales de médecine,* publish reports on the professional and medical situation in the United States and other countries.[22]

In the article, which was published in the *Annales médico-psychologiques,* one of the very first French psychiatry journals, de la Sagra commented upon the statistics and the differentials obtained between black and white insanity in the South and the North. De la Sagra reported the numerical differences between the numbers of white and black individuals classified as insane, reporting the results as "remarkable" and "worthy of attention," specifically when one "looks precisely at the insane persons who belong to the categories of the free people of color and to the slaves." De la Sagra remarked with amazement that "the number of lunatics among the first category [free] is considerably greater than among the second category [enslaved], to the extent that one can never find or even imagine a similar situation in Europe." De la Sagra then announced that he intended to seek the causes of this madness among free Blacks.

The rhetoric used by de la Sagra is worthy of note, in that he was commenting upon a social context different from his own, from his position as an outsider who observed "from afar" the medical and institutional practices in the United States. De la Sagra questioned the accuracy of the numbers in the southern states based on his suspicion of "some omissions on the part of the masters (which would lead us to believe that the number of lunatics is even greater than what transpires from the census)." According to de la Sagra, the census returns could not be the result of systemic miscalculations, because "no government or local government has any vested interest in pretending that the country is awash with idiots and imbeciles, whether in the white race or the African race." De la Sagra affirmed that even a proslavery government could have nothing to gain from increasing the numbers of lunatics within its territory.

He concluded that the causes of madness in the United States had multiple origins, arguing that "it is the search for these causes and the study of these conditions that have put me on the path of the results that I present today, and which are only part of a larger work that will include the social status of people of color, free and emancipated, in terms of their education, their vices and their criminality, prostitution in women, drunkenness among men, misery amongst all, etc." De la Sagra added that "the figures concerning the number of lunatics, among men of color, provide remarkable data, which should be compared with the conditions of their existence in the United States," thus arguing that maybe the disproportion between the numbers of enslaved and free Blacks had nothing to do with slavery but with the social environment in which free black people lived.

According to de la Sagra, free black individuals were the victims of "disdain and scorn, by the effect of a severe prejudice against them." De la Sagra argued that this disdain and scorn prevailed "among the white class of the northern states of the Confederation." Free black individuals also suffered from the "almost complete lack of public amusements in this country of strict puritanism" and underwent a state of "frequent religious excitation in Methodist meetings and gatherings of other sects." More importantly, de la Sagra thought that the prevalence of insanity in the United States was due to certain American behaviors and customs, such as "religious exaltation and the absence of distractions, combined with the cerebral commotion resulting from the prevailing industrial mania and the fever for commerce, which is observed to such a high degree among the Americans." To him, "these causes, . . . can help explain the large number of lunatics which also exist among the Whites of the northern states, a number which, though less than that of free people of color, is, however, very considerable." He concluded his remarks by saying, "Until now, no country in Europe has offered such high ratios," which, to him, further proved that the problem was national and not only due to slavery.[23]

De la Sagra's argument was radically opposed both to Jarvis's arguments and to the proslavery rhetoric that naturalized the social fact of madness by ascribing it to the "essence" of the black race. De la Sagra further called for a program of studies on the social conditions of people of color in the United States. Thus, the census of 1840 opened up a whole series of questions among essayists, philosophers, and doctors trying to understand this recrudescence of madness among Blacks in the North. Furthermore, de la Sagra did not make a distinction between Blacks and Whites but among individual "Americans," who were subject to "industrial mania and the fever for commerce," "religious exaltation," and "puritanism," any or all of which would provoke madness, while among Europeans, madness had never "offered such high ratios." His reading of the statistical results was therefore profoundly different from that of American doctors from either the North or the South, because he did not rely on the racial frameworks previously established in American history. In addition, de la Sagra explained the insanity of people of color as a result of the disdain and scorn of Whites, thus paying more attention to the social and psychological causes, resulting from racial prejudice, in the manifestation of madness than to biological notions—the latter being the crux of the arguments of the southern and northern physicians in the United States during the same time period.

Although Ramon de la Sagra published his paper in a French academic journal for a Francophone audience only, it is important to highlight his contribution, since it shows that the arguments about the U.S. census were not considered by physicians and policymakers only in the United States but also circulated in Europe as well. His arguments further reveal the many transnational debates on the politicization of statistics on insanity in the nineteenth century. This has not been noted previously in relation to the 1840 census controversy, since historians have focused solely on American contributions to the debate.

The most flamboyant and determined denunciation of both the statistics and Calhoun's prose was made by James McCune Smith, one of the first black doctors, who was living in New York at the time. In January 1844, Smith published an article in which he responded with great bitterness to the *Southern Literary Messenger* piece, stating that "freedom has not made us [Blacks] mad; it has strengthened our minds by throwing us upon our own resources and has bound us to American institutions with a tenacity which nothing but death can overcome."[24]

Smith's denunciation was directly linked to his self-defined position as the spokesperson for free Blacks in the North. Three months after the publication of this first article, on Friday May 3, 1844, Smith attended a public meeting at the Zion church in New York, which had been organized by the Reverend Henry H. Garnet, a prominent spokesperson in the free Black community. The meeting was advertised as follows: "Fellow citizens! will you suffer yourselves to be branded by a bigoted slaveholder, as being 'invariably sunk into vice and pauperism,' accompanied by the bodily and mental inflictions incident thereto . . . , without a murmur, without a denial? Then let every man and woman attend en masse. The colored citizens of Brooklyn, Williamsburg, and Newark are respectfully invited to attend."

The meeting proved to be a success. The *New York Herald* reported that "at 8 o'clock, the church (which is a neat and simple edifice) was crowded to excess with 'the gentlemen of color,' and the galleries were filled to overflowing with the choicest specimens of the 'fair portion of creation,' who seemed much interested in the emancipation of their 'sable' brothers of the South."[25] The meeting concluded with a vote on a memorial to be presented to Congress to oppose Calhoun's reading of the statistics. The memorialists pointed out that "in asserting the existence of free colored persons insane, blind, deaf and dumb in certain towns in the free states, in which towns, it appears by the same census of 1840, there are no free colored persons whatever of any condition." They thus asked for the 1840 census to be "re-examined, and so far as possible, corrected and, in the Department of State, in order that the head of that Department may have facts upon which to found his arguments."

Although this episode has been overlooked by previous contributions to the history of the U.S. census, it demonstrates that the black community in New York, whose members included Smith, was deeply concerned about the release of the U.S. census returns in 1840 and fought vigorously and collectively against their circulation, especially because these statistics were used to support arguments that questioned their legitimate claims to freedom and emancipation. Indeed, Smith and Garnet were two of the most significant and influential abolitionists in the American Anti-Slavery Society of the 1840s and 1850s.[26] Their opposition to the census figures is not just an indication that free black New Yorkers resented white supremacists' analyses of the 1840 census; it also demonstrates that they were aware that Calhoun and proslavery apologists could use the census figures as a political tool against the abolitionist movement itself, by brandishing the argument that freedom caused insanity in black bodies. The controversy over the 1840 census was therefore a watershed moment in the politicization of the black psyche, because of its potential implications for emancipation movements.

Despite the refutations, the 1840 statistics continued to spread their influence over even the reception of the 1850 census, the results of which came to be seen as proof, to southern journalists, that the 1840 census results were correct. In September 1851, the *Charleston Mercury* published an article in which data from the 1840 census was compared to data from the 1850 census. Although "the tables of 1850 are not yet published," the article explained, "some of the returns have been ascertained sufficiently to confirm the results obtained from those of 1840. . . . These details furnish materials for ample speculation to the physiologist, the moralist and the statesman. They touch the great problem which philanthropists, not ranting enthusiasts or reckless theorists, but sound and humane thinkers, study with painful solicitude: what is the destiny of this race, morally and physically, in any state but that of slavery."[27]

The article continued, espousing the proslavery point of view: "In this country, all the evidence goes to show that freedom has been to them, morally and physically, a curse instead of a blessing; that it has degraded instead of elevating them socially, weakened their physical powers, and wasted their energy as a race. On this continent, with society as now organized, every slave liberated is one more added to a mass of inevitable suffering and predestined decay—a fact which develops itself more and more strongly every day." Such was the conclusion of this newspaper, highlighting for us today that the impact of the 1840 statistics did not come to an end in the 1840s.

In fact, the statistics regained popularity throughout the 1850s, as sectionalist tensions rose due to major political changes. The Mexican Cession (1848) was partly responsible for the rise of tensions between northern and southern states. With the Treaty of Guadalupe Hidalgo, Mexico ceded more than 525,000 square miles of territory to the United States, which reignited the slavery issue.[28] The Wilmot Proviso, which was designed to eliminate slavery within the land acquired as a result of the Mexican War, was unsuccessful in Congress. Nonetheless, it heightened tensions between northerners, who feared the addition of slave territory, and southerners, who saw the proposal as an attack on their way of life.[29] Parallel to these national debates over sectional balance, abolitionist groups and organizations in the North, such as the American Anti-Slavery Society, which had been founded in the 1830s, gained remarkable momentum in such places as Boston and New York.[30] In retaliation, the major presses and newspapers of the "cotton kingdom" published editorials against abolitionism and any potential restrictions on slavery.[31]

In this context, proslavery southern physicians such as James D. Barkdull sought to legitimize slavery by any means necessary. Barkdull, who graduated from the Medical College of Louisiana in 1854 and shortly thereafter became a physician at the state hospital at Jackson, Louisiana, explained in 1858 that black individuals' exemption from insanity in the South was "due to their situation, the protection the law guarantees to them, the restraint of a mild state of servitude, the freedom from anxiety respecting their present and future wants, the withholding (in great degree) of spirituous and drugged liquors, and other forms of excess into which the free negroes plunge in this and all other countries, to the utter ruin of mind, body, and estate."

"As far as my knowledge extends in the surrounding parishes," he further explained, "I have never seen a single case of insanity in this State, or Mississippi, where I practiced medicine for several years. But, on the contrary, it is also my experience, that free negroes, from the before-mentioned and other causes unnecessary to detail, are peculiarly predisposed to insanity."[32]

Barkdull's claims were facilitated by the circulation of the 1840 statistics on insanity, which had also popularized the chain of causality between freedom and the madness affecting black individuals. In 1854, a similar claim was made by journalists from the *Washington Sentinel*. Quoting the 1840 census returns on insanity, they argued that "the Southern slave is infinitely better cared for and more comfortable than the free colored population of the Southern States."[33]

The statistics even found their way past the mid-1850s. In "Facts Worth Noticing," an article published by the *Macon Weekly Telegraph* in Georgia, the authors examined the state of "the physiological deterioration of the free blacks, particularly in the non-slaveholding States of the Republic." Relying on the 1850 census results, they maintained that the 1840 census results were accurate, despite the memorials that had been sent to Congress: "It will be seen by the compendium of the U.S. census for 1850, compiled from official documents by Professor De Bow, superintendent of the Census Bureau, and published by the authority of Congress in 1854, that after a thorough scrutiny by the government, the authenticity of the census, so unfavorable to the physical and sanitary condition of the free Blacks of the North, is fully established."[34] By 1853, J. C. G. Kennedy had been replaced as superintendent clerk of the U.S. census by none other than James Dunwoody Brownson De Bow, an influential southern publisher and editor of *De Bow's Review.*

In 1856, *Hunt's Merchants' Magazine and Commercial Review,* a prominent New York journal, published an article that summarized the results of the latest census. A major part of this short essay concerned the figures for insanity affecting black individuals in 1850 and their comparison with figures from 1840. The article indicated that for "all classes, the mean of the last three censuses shows one affected person to every 957 whites in the slaveholding states, and one to 1,060 in the other states; one to every 1,444 colored in the slaveholding states and one to 503 in the non-slaveholding." All in all, the author of the article, L. Woodruff, tried to demonstrate that the results obtained in 1850 remained the same as those of 1840, especially when one compared the averages. "This singular disproportion in the number of free colored and slave deaf, dumb, blind, etc. is observable throughout previous censuses," explained Woodruff, quoting Secretary of State Calhoun.[35] More than fifteen years after their first publication, and despite the efforts of black residents of New York and of James McCune Smith to disavow and condemn the document, the statistics on insanity from the 1840 and 1850 censuses were still viewed as authentic proof, reflecting the mental situation of free black individuals in the North.

One year later, in 1857, an article entitled "Black and White Insanity" was published in the *Charleston Mercury.* The data from the article was itself reprinted from an article published in *Hall's Journal of Health* during the same year, in which the insanity of black northerners was attributed to their freedom. Free black individuals from the North were described as having their minds eaten out by "the struggle and anxiety for daily bread." Enslaved people were described by the author as having "no such anxieties," because "their lives are merrier than those of their masters; they know that bread would be given to them, and their water shall be sure; and having food . . . they are therewith content, measurably." According to the author, "the mass of slaves in our country assent to the religious sentiments either by practice, profession, or proclivity and have learned in whatsoever state they are, therewith to be content."

"There can be no doubt that with other aids, the burden of slavery is comparatively light to them," argued the author, who then quoted "the lively song on the levee, in New Orleans," which was "the song of the slave" and "helped them to work easy." According to the author, enslaved people's use of music was very different from the customs of Irish laborers, who were described as more unhappy than the enslaved, since "we never heard a note of music from [them] in ten years."[36]

The southern journalists' accusatory rhetoric was no coincidence, considering the increasing political conflict taking place on a large scale between abolitionists in the North and the white proslavery elite in the South. The *Dred Scott* case had torn the country in half over the issue of slavery in 1857, which was the same year as the publication of the article in the *Charleston Mercury*. Dred Scott was an enslaved man whose enslavers had taken him from his plantation in Missouri to Illinois, where slavery was illegal. When he was later brought back to Missouri, Scott sued for his freedom in court, claiming that his residency in Illinois had automatically freed him and that he was legally no longer enslaved. The Supreme Court, which issued a 7–2 decision against Scott, was widely discussed in the northern press, and in the South as well, where southerners rejoiced over the Supreme Court justices' opinions.

In 1859, the *Christian Examiner* decided to debunk the arguments and claims concerning the 1850 census by publishing an article by the Reverend James Freeman Clarke. Clarke's article denounced the figures, saying that they "were consummate liars, and that, in many of the localities given, the insane colored people existed only in the figures of the census. It was the census that was insane, and not the colored people." Furthermore, Clarke attacked De Bow (who became the superintendent of the Census Bureau in 1853, after Joseph C. G. Kennedy, who served from 1850 to 1853) for presenting false figures that clearly supported proslavery arguments, thus repeating the mistakes of 1840: "Whether similar blunders, all on the side of slavery may not have been committed in preparing the tables of 1850, we know not; but we cannot rely fully on the fairness of statement in one like Mr. De Bow, whose principal business in life, down to the time that he was appointed Superintendent of the Census . . . was editing a magazine of the most proslavery proclivities, and which he still continues to edit."[37] Indeed, even though Joseph C. G. Kennedy was superintendent of the Census Bureau at the time of the planning the 1850 census and during its data collection, De Bow managed the last steps of the census's completion, from 1853 to 1855, publishing the census results and producing statistical reports on the census returns.

A few months later, in 1860, the *American Journal of Insanity* published a short report written by Robley Dunglison, an English physician who had moved to America to join the first faculty of the University of Virginia. Dunglison stipulated that despite the "extreme unreliability of the statistics presented," one could see that "insanity prevails to a greater extent among the white and free colored population than among the slaves," and that insanity affecting black individuals was especially due to "care and anxiety, and from intemperance and other excesses," which shows the survival of the argument that freedom was a cause of madness, more than twenty years after the publication of the first census returns.[38]

Dunglison's use of these statistics appeared on the eve of the Civil War, when sectional tensions had never been more intense. A violent conflict over the legality of slavery started in the proposed state of Kansas, between antislavery Free-Staters and proslavery "border ruffians" from Missouri.[39] Historians of the period often refer to the conflict, which spanned the years 1854 to 1859, as a prelude to the Civil War, and it was extensively discussed by the local and national press in all the states of the Union.[40] The Republican Party emerged in 1854 to combat the extension of slavery into the Western territories and consisted mostly of northern professionals. Furthermore, debates over popular sovereignty intensified on the subject of whether the territories beyond the Western frontier, which were about to join the Union, should prohibit or permit slavery. The doctrine of popular sovereignty was overwhelmingly supported in the southern states, where the white proslavery elite promoted the idea that residents of a territory, and not the federal government, should be allowed to decide on slavery within their borders.[41] These debates and conflicts further intensified the sectional divide over slavery.

The argument that freedom was a cause of insanity gained credence in the Reconstruction era, more than thirty years after the original publication of the 1840 census statistics. For example, in 1871, a couple of years after the end of the Civil War, the *Weekly Louisianian,* a New Orleans newspaper, published an article in which census data was quoted to inform the readers that freedmen and freedwomen suffered from insanity at a much higher rate than white southerners.[42] Yet, after 1865, in the Reconstruction context, commentators now quoted the insanity statistics in support of a return to slavery and against newly acquired black civil rights. The reading of the statistics by southern commentators had therefore slightly shifted with the advent of the Civil War. The

behavior of free black individuals in the northern states was no longer scrutinized. Now, southern physicians and members of the white political elite from
the former Confederate states turned to the population of freedwomen and
freedmen in order to argue that emancipation had rendered them unfit for
work and mentally unstable.

This impugning of emancipation as the main cause of insanity was also
brought up by professors of medicine in Louisiana in the late 1880s, thus showing that the statistics, and what might be termed the "freedom cause" of insanity, soon found their way into medical classrooms. In the South, the Medical
College of Louisiana, founded in 1834 (known as the Medical Department of
the University of Louisiana after the late 1840s), played a significant role in the
rediscovery of these statistics and the supposed correlation between freedom
and insanity among black individuals. In his 1889 medical lecture at the eleventh annual session of the Louisiana State Medical Society in New Orleans, a
professor at the Medical College of Louisiana and former Confederate officer,
Joseph Jones, made a reference to the significant numbers of black patients in
asylums in the South, attributing their insanity to "political excitement." Using
examples of cases of insanity affecting Blacks from the New Orleans Charity
Hospital, Jones defined "political excitement" as similar to "religious excitement," affirming it to be provoked by "hereditary or congenital imperfections
of the nervous system" as well as by "chronic alcoholism and masturbation."
To Jones, "political excitement and certain political and race changes, such as
those wrought by the great American civil war of 1861–1865," were the cause of
his black patients' mental afflictions, thus provoking a "demoniacal" change in
their mental state.[43]

Jones's argument also demonstrates that the statistics and the "freedom
cause" found a new place in the political economy of the South after the Civil
War. In the New South, the Redeemers formed political coalitions in the southern states, which sought to regain political power and enforce white supremacy.[44] Many white southerners managed to overthrow or defeat Republicans
after Reconstruction and thereby established a long-term Democratic domi-
nance over southern institutions. In the 1870s, these new local governments
passed measures such as the black codes that effectively blocked black suffrage, thus marking the end of Reconstruction. They also facilitated the enforcement of measures such as sharecropping and debt peonage on behalf of
white landowners who sought to appropriate the work potential of freedmen
and freedwomen.[45]

By developing a medical argument in this way, Jones was intentionally pointing a finger at the 1863 Emancipation Proclamation, effectively accusing it of directly impacting the health and moral character of newly freed individuals, who he claimed were not able to handle the new era of freedom. Jones therefore fully participated in the Redeemers' ideology, which consisted in restoring a moral, social, and political order based on white supremacy. Jones also made the argument that while the Reconstruction era had durably impacted the health and morality of formerly enslaved people, white southerners and former Confederate officers were not affected by the same severe change in their mental condition. To Jones, "the consciousness in the justice of the cause for which their lives and fortunes were risked[,] their brave . . . nature[,] the physical development and perfection of the men and women of the Southern States" as well as "the four years of incessant marching, entrenching and fighting which characterized the campaigns of the Southern army during the struggle (1861–1865)," inured the soldiers to hardship, "hard work, frugal and scant meals, and educated their minds to face, without a murmur, disease, disaster and death." While "the heroic struggle tried the hearts of the entire male population of the Southern States in the fierce fires of battle and prepared them to struggle manfully with subsequent degradation resulting from defeat," black men and women were doomed to insanity, due to their new political and moral condition.[46] Jones's double-edged argument thus further affirmed the supposed rise of madness among black populations while highlighting the white man's moral and mental qualities after Reconstruction.

Insanity in the black population was still being discussed in the 1890s in relation to emancipation and the acquisition of civil rights. In 1890, the *Plaindealer,* an African American newspaper in Detroit, Michigan, published an article saying that insanity was becoming "an alarming future in the course of present civilization."

"Until recently the Afro Americans were almost exempt from its influence," the paper stated, "but now having entered into the energy and restlessness of the present age, they too are becoming subjects of dementia."[47] The freedmen and freedwomen were thus seen as having just entered a state of civilization— some of them had experienced the effect of relocating to cities after leaving the plantations, which, according to the author, did not necessarily entail better living conditions for them. This article can be read as a statement of concern for the mental health of black citizens as they made the transition into free society and faced a new range of discriminations from white Americans.

More than thirty years after the Civil War, freedom was still discussed in southern medical circles as a cause of insanity for freedmen and their descendants. In 1900, J. Addison Hodges, a physician from Richmond, Virginia, read a paper before the American Medico-Psychological Association on "The Effect of Freedom upon the Physical and Psychological Development of the Negro," in which he observed that the number of black individuals classified as insane had drastically increased since 1865 in the state of Virginia. Hodges quoted census results from 1800, 1840, 1860, 1880, and 1890 to support his case, while also quoting his colleague from South Carolina, Dr. Powell, who argued that "there has been a radical change in the susceptibility to certain diseases, notably insanity, phthisis and similar maladies in this class of our population, from which they were almost entirely exempt up to 1867." According to Hodges, under slavery, enslaved people's "habits of life were regular, their food and clothing were substantial and sufficient as a rule, and the edict of their masters restrained them from promiscuous excesses and the baneful influences of unrestricted indulgences."

"By other authorities it has been claimed that the increase of insanity among the negroes in Virginia has been for 25 years at the rate of 100, or more, per cent, every ten years," wrote Hodges, who was eager to prove that "the negro race is especially liable to certain forms of nervous diseases," especially after 1865 and the Civil War.[48]

How can one explain the recrudescence of the "freedom cause," or freedom causality factor, tying up madness with freedom, more than fifty years after the publication of the 1840 census? Were the words of James Barkdull, Joseph Jones, and J. Addison Hodges, among others, isolated acts or were they part of a consistent medical line of reasoning?

In many respects, their words were not freak occurrences. Reconstruction had actively marked the southern political and collective imagination, and it was seen as a disastrous and nightmarish moment, a debacle, by white southerners, who had lost control of their territories to the Union.[49] Their arguments present the specificity of having been written during a period when racial and social hierarchies had been shattered in the southern states. They reacted bitterly to social changes that they saw as brutal and unfair. Until the 1860s, white southerners had mobilized the argument of madness affecting black populations to raise the threatening specter of a racial dystopia in the South, trying to dissuade abolitionists from pushing their movement forward by announcing that this would further weaken vulnerable Whites in the face of what they called hordes of mad and dangerous black men and women, and that black individuals also would suffer as a result. Then, after emancipation, freedom as a causality factor was launched on a new trajectory. It was quickly taken up by southern physicians hoping to regain control of the rhetorical territory by marshaling the medicalization of madness along with nostalgia for an antebellum golden age. The signing of the Emancipation Proclamation in 1863 thus crystallized in a new way the fears of physicians and statesmen, giving rise to a new medical narrative that bent itself according to the political context.

Thus, medical explanations that linked freedom and madness did not fade out in the context of the great emancipation. Quite to the contrary, these medical explanations circulated in the words and writings of professors and students from the Medical College of Louisiana, such as Joseph Jones and James D. Barkdull; physicians from Virginia, such as J. Addison Hodges and Robley Dunglinson; and journalists whose opinions were featured in the *Washington Sentinel* (District of Columbia), the *Weekly Louisianian* (New Orleans), the *Macon Weekly Telegraph* (Georgia), or the *Charleston Mercury* (South Carolina) over a prolonged period of time, from the 1850s to the 1890s. They also circulated in the North and abroad, as they were cited by political commentators in the *Plaindealer* or *Hunt's Merchants' Magazine,* which shows that these theories gained much popularity and crossed regional and national boundaries.

Those who refuted the credibility of the censuses and the statistical claims arising from them were not only white northern physicians but also foreign commentators such as Ramón de la Sagra and black residents of New York such as James McCune Smith. The actions of Smith and his circle are especially interesting to highlight, since their positions have often been overlooked in the literature. Their interventions reveal to us today that these statistics on madness encountered great resistance because they were seen by free men and women of color in New York as potential threats to black freedom.

Despite their refutations, however, the arguments linking freedom and emancipation continued to circulate and were transformed over time to fit the new post–Civil War political context, after slavery had been abolished. It was no longer a question of saying that the longer the black individuals had been freed, the more mentally ill they were, but rather of insisting on the exponential growth of madness affecting black populations since enslaved people had become freedmen, therefore initiating a broader medical-political commentary on the topics of civil rights and mental soundness. The next chapters will examine how this medical-political commentary on civil rights and insanity came to be applied in various southern asylums and hospitals treating black patients from the 1860s onward, thus showing how these theories were transformed into concrete and performative racialist treatments that shaped the practices of southern physicians in the long term.

3

THE OPENING OF PSYCHIATRIC
INSTITUTIONS FOR BLACK PATIENTS
IN THE SOUTH, 1860–1880

I know what the caged bird feels, alas!
When the sun is bright on the upland slopes;
When the wind stirs soft through the springing grass,
And the river flows like a stream of glass;
When the first bird sings and the first bud opes,
And the faint perfume from its chalice steals—
I know what the caged bird feels!

—PAUL LAURENCE DUNBAR, "Sympathy" (1899)

In March 1877, toward the end of the Reconstruction era, Robert F. Baldwin, the director of the Western Lunatic Asylum in Staunton, Virginia, and former physician in the Confederate army, received a letter from Martin Scott, who was a professor at the Medical College of Virginia in Richmond. Scott's questions flowed in quick succession over three separate sheets, urging Baldwin to take up his pen to give speedy reply. Quoting the previous census returns, Scott wanted Baldwin to send him the admissions statistics from the Central Lunatic Asylum for Colored Insane at Howard's Grove, near Richmond (soon to move to Petersburg and later renamed the Central State Hospital), which had opened in Virginia eight years previously, in order to compare them to the national average. Scott was particularly worried about the spread of madness in the Commonwealth of Virginia more than ten years after the Civil War.

"In your opinion has Emancipation increased the numbers of insane negroes? Had the war and its results increased the number of insane whites in Virginia?" asked Scott, eager to know more about Baldwin's understanding of epidemiological links between emancipation and madness. Apologizing for speaking so directly to his colleague, Scott explained that he was seized with a "curiosity to know if there has not been an increase in the number of insane negroes, ratio of insane, since the war and as a consequence of the delights of freedom," a curiosity that could only be satisfied by the answers of Dr. Baldwin, a renowned physician in the South, who had trained at the prestigious University of Pennsylvania.[1]

Scott was a former Confederate physician, and his motives for obtaining the admissions statistics were chiefly political, as he sought scientific proof of insanity affecting Blacks in order to avenge, at least in spirit, the Confederate defeat.[2] But in the wake of his missive, his initial curiosity soon turned to anger as he tried to understand the rapid expansion of madness in Virginia in light of what he saw as the disastrous southern political situation: "I want the Yankees to have the satisfaction of knowing how much evil they have brought upon Virginia without whose aid that self-satisfied, self-glorifying people would still be under British rule," wrote Scott. He added that he "desires them to know that not only have they brought ruin upon her people but have consigned so many to her mad-house . . . but also that their peculiar pets can't stand the cons and responsibilities of freedom."

Scott saw a causal link between, on the one hand, the marked increase in the madness of Blacks and Whites in the state and, on the other, the military occupation of approximately one hundred southern towns and cities immediately after the Civil War, which white southerners had to bear and which, at the same time, precipitated the collapse of the southern order.[3] Indeed, Scott questioned the alleged increase of madness the better to assert it; he hoped to receive a response from Baldwin confirming his first intuition, showing that black individuals had become particularly susceptible to madness as a consequence of being freed.[4]

At the end of Reconstruction, the spread of madness was thus perceived in the South as the result of a large-scale political and social dysfunction, for which northerners were largely responsible. Southerners such as Scott resented northern policy because it promoted Unionism, which they saw as a pattern of uniformization that would strip seceding states of their "way of life."[5] Indeed,

Radical Republicans in Congress after 1865 aimed to curtail the rights of former Confederate southerners who had opposed Unionism, introducing legislation such as the Wade-Davis Bill of 1864, which forced former Confederate soldiers and supporters to swear they had never supported the Confederacy—an oath referred to as the Ironclad Oath—as a way of preventing them from being politically active.[6] Although the bill was pocket vetoed by Abraham Lincoln and never took effect, it caused waves of outrage in the South and exacerbated ex-Confederate supporters' anger.

Yet Reconstruction policies did not merely target southern political power; they aimed to protect the well-being of freedmen and freedwomen with provisions such as the creation of the Freedmen's Bureau. Many episodes of racial violence took place in the early stages of Reconstruction in response to the promise of extending black civil rights. In May 1866, in Memphis, mobs of white residents and policemen rampaged through black neighborhoods, killing forty-six freedmen and freedwomen and burning down ninety-one homes, four churches, and eight schools (every black church and school) in the black community.[7] A couple of months later, in July 1866, a mob of white rioters attacked peaceful black protesters who had organized a demonstration in New Orleans to obtain voting rights. Approximately fifty marchers were killed before federal troops, who were stationed in New Orleans, could suppress the riot and jail the white insurgents.

Such events strengthened even further the case of Radical Republicans, who called for further protective measures for freedmen, such as military districts and oversights in some states, as well as the Fourteenth Amendment, which granted full citizenship to formerly enslaved people after 1868.[8] Nonetheless, the late 1860s and the 1870s continued to be the theater of many other episodes of racial violence against black civilians, such as the St. Landry massacre in Louisiana (1868), the Meridian race riot in Mississippi (1871), the Colfax massacre in Louisiana (1873), and the Hamburg massacre in South Carolina (1876).[9] In many ways, Scott's violent rhetoric toward northerners and formerly enslaved people mirrors this broader southern context of white violence against black individuals.

By sending this letter, Scott also sought to link the admissions statistics to a more recent event: the 1869 opening of the Central Lunatic Asylum, the first asylum for black patients in Virginia. "Virginia has recently established I believe a negro insane asylum. . . . Was this rendered necessary by the increase of her negro insane, or as a matter of caste? Or both? Do you receive negro insane in your institution? How does the percentage of 'cure' of the two races compare?" asked Scott, trying to make sense of the founding of this new institution.

Were this epistolary exchange an isolated incident, it would be merely anecdotal. However, it takes on a whole new dimension when analyzed in relation to the moral economy of the South in which it occurred. What were the opinions of southern Whites and black elites of the state about this new institution? What other, similar institutions emerged? How were these new racialized medical spaces organized?[10] Scott's words show that the circulation of statistics on insanity affecting black individuals created anxiety among white physicians, who were concerned that additional institutions for black patients classified as insane would be required in Virginia and would consequently need funding. This led to the fear that white southerners would have to pay for the institutionalization of black patients, for whom they felt no solidarity, especially in the context of political insurgency against Republicans and Unionism.

Scott's use of these federal statistics concerning madness, like the other uses outlined in chapter 2, were tied to local debates on race, power, and pathology in the South, even long after the 1840 census controversy. Furthermore, Scott's political use of these statistics on insanity unveils how the arguments tying together madness and emancipation were used by southern physicians in the immediate post–Civil War Reconstruction era to prove that formerly enslaved people were being diagnosed with insanity, a condition that was thought to have been caused by their new status as freedmen and freedwomen.

This chapter sheds light on the context of the opening of two asylums hosting only black patients: the Central Lunatic Asylum and the Eastern North Carolina Insane Asylum, founded in Goldsboro, North Carolina, in 1880. It also examines segregated state institutions in Louisiana that admitted black patients in separate wings, such as the Central Louisiana State Hospital, opened in Pineville in 1902.[11] The opening of these institutions in three southern states sparked unprecedented economic and therapeutic debates in the New South, and studying them provides answers to several questions. To begin, we must understand the issues of building hospitals and asylums for black patients, which were rare in the United States at that time. In this respect, the Central Lunatic Asylum for Colored Insane, opened in 1869, during Reconstruction, presents a uniquely interesting case, being the oldest hospital for black patients only in the United States.[12] As such, it represents the architectural and management model upon which other black hospitals would later be founded. Despite the historic importance of the Central Lunatic Asylum, few works have examined the conditions and debates that led to its opening, or the preponderant role that such an institution for black patients in the South could play, twenty years after the Civil War.[13]

The hospital at Goldsboro, North Carolina, has seldom been the subject of research, despite the fact it was the second black psychiatric asylum to open in the South, in 1880.[14] The Central Louisiana State Hospital in Pineville is a useful case study when looking into segregated hospitals starting in the 1900s. This hospital offers a unique opportunity for the study of the treatment of black patients in psychiatric institutions in the nineteenth century because it hosted both black and white patients in separate wards and thus provides points of comparison in terms of treatments and facilities.

Studying the ways in which racialized patients across these three states were treated in public institutions provides a more representative portrait of the racialized southern medical context than restricting oneself to a single location. I also will be looking at the hospital as a possible place of resistance for black patients, as the funding of asylums was supported by the first black legislators elected in Virginia during Reconstruction. Did the building of asylums for black individuals meet white economic resistance, and what does it teach us about the medical treatments of black patients in the South?

As we saw in chapter 1, no systematic legislation regulated the treatment of enslaved people experiencing mental illness in the antebellum South, but a few institutions could, against payment, receive enslaved people, who were then placed in the same wings as Whites. A. H. Witmer, in an article dating from 1891, mentions the opening of the first asylum for black patients in Mississippi, the Mississippi State Hospital, at the initiative of its director, Dr. A. D. Williamson. In 1858, Williamson had submitted a report to the governor of his state, William McWillie, to inform him of the need to take into account the fate of black patients classified as insane, having previously petitioned Charles H. Nichols, director of the Government Hospital for the Insane, in Washington, DC, to do the same, in 1855.[15] Witmer pointed out, however, that these initiatives did not involve the construction of specific buildings for black individuals.

The systematic institutionalization of black patients in significant numbers, in an institution dedicated to them, began in the 1870s, in Virginia. Previously, admissions had increased in the few asylums that accepted black patients, especially in Virginia. Yet, at the Eastern Lunatic Asylum at Williamsburg, also in Virginia, local medical authorities had begun to question the notion of racial integration.[16] Likewise, during the 1860s, doctors in the South Carolina Lunatic Asylum argued that integration had a negative impact on the health of Whites interned in the same institution. This anti-integrationist vision was shared by both southern and northern physicians. Thomas Kirkbride, a physician at the Pennsylvania Hospital, affirmed in 1855 that "the idea of mixing up all colors and classes . . . is not what is wanted in our hospital for the insane," condemning racial integration in these asylums.[17]

Kirkbride's antebellum advocacy of racial segregation in medical institutions in Philadelphia parallels the history of northern segregation in the era of gradual emancipation. Historians of the nineteenth century have long documented how northerners, even though slavery had vanished from their social space, still held a deep racialist ideology that permeated their political and economic life. Historian Margot Minardi has demonstrated how the history of slavery in Massachusetts and New England was hidden in plain sight in a form of collective amnesia that facilitated public opposition to southern slavery, before being recovered by memorializing attempts in recent years.[18]

Similarly, historian Joanne Pope Melish has shown how people of color in New England suffered from social invisibility after the 1820s, precisely when northern critics chose to focus on southern slavery as the locus of evil.[19] In this idealized narrative, northerners depicted themselves as representing the fortress of American liberty, even though, as historian Leon Litwack has revealed, people of color often experienced discrimination and prejudice in economic and political life in free New England.[20] As Minardi has demonstrated, for instance, it was not uncommon for northern physicians to view black bodies as biologically different from white bodies, even in the same political and social spaces where slavery had been abolished.

In Virginia, the creation of the first asylum for black patients only, which was founded in 1869 and opened in 1870, owed its success to the mobilization of the newly elected black legislators between 1865 and 1877, during Reconstruction.[21] The Central Lunatic Asylum was the first institution opened only for Blacks in the New South.[22] Far from being conceived from the outset as an instrument of social control—as is often argued in more general works on the functioning of mental asylums in the nineteenth century—this asylum was first conceived by the Republican Virginia Assembly members as a social welfare institution to help the destitute or otherwise vulnerable black population in Virginia.[23]

In the Reconstruction era, black men in the southern states gained the vote long before the Jim Crow laws were passed (after 1877) and confiscated the fruits of their latest democratic advances.[24] During this short, temporary window after the war, several black lawmakers, including Matt Clark, Robert Norton, Caesar Perkins, and Burwell Toler, were elected in Virginia. Norton and Clark were appointed to the Committee on Asylums and Prisons, which ruled on the creation of an asylum for black patients in 1868. Following this first victory, other mobilizations ensued. One of the first parliamentary battles of Clark, a native of Halifax County who was elected to the Virginia House of Delegates, was to submit and defend a resolution that was intended to support the improvement of living conditions of Central Lunatic Asylum patients.

Perkins, elected in 1869 and a native of Buckingham County, was one of the black legislators who, in 1888, voted to increase grants for the asylum and for state educational institutions for black individuals, such as the State Female Normal School (later renamed Longwood University, in Farmville, Virginia). Perkins was known for his fight for the advancement of education and public services for black people. Born enslaved, he had participated locally in organizing the Freedmen's Bureau and the Bureau of Refugees after the war and in 1868 had bought land in his home county in order to set up a church and a school for black children. The mobilizations for the creation of schools and the Central Lunatic Asylum thus followed the same logic: to grant black citizens the same access to social welfare and education as white citizens already had. These were the first mobilizations at the heart of the program of local black elites during the Reconstruction era.[25]

Black legislators, however, opposed the segregation that the new asylum represented, fearing that it would lead to inequality and inadequate treatment of the black population compared to what was offered at the asylums for Whites. On the other hand, for the newly elected black Virginia legislators, the asylum for black patients symbolized obvious scientific and social progress. For a start, it allowed the black population to cross the portals of a medical institution, which was seen as the paragon of modernity by physicians and lay circles at the time. However, the black legislators' vision was not realized in practice, as the asylum failed even early on to provide adequate therapeutic betterment for its black patients. Instead, it was transformed into a punitive, penitentiary-style institution, which functioned with an all-white staff in the nineteenth and early twentieth centuries.

The asylum was also thought to be a new form of public assistance for the black poor, since it would come to the aid of those who were sick but also of widows, orphans, and old men, not all of whom were necessarily mentally ill and all of whom were admitted after 1870.[26] In the nineteenth century, the asylum system in the whole of the United States rose from the need for public assistance at the local level. The families of most mentally ill antebellum Americans could not afford to care for them, and so those family members became public wards of the town, county, or state. As David Rothman shows in his authoritative account, supporters of the movement for federal assistance for asylum building during the Jacksonian era justified their demands with the argument that many states, counties, and towns were having trouble funding the care of their indigents. At the same time, the development of asylums reinforced moral and public order and was a way of restoring the lost virtue of colonial rule.[27]

As historian Michael B. Katz has shown, "public relief is an American tradition with roots firmly planted in the colonial period," although in the antebellum South there was less political willingness locally to provide public assistance to the mentally ill.[28] Indeed, writing about the rise of poorhouses and asylums in the early 1800s, historian David Wagner concludes that "some regions, such as the Southern states, provided little or no social welfare of any type (indoor or outdoor relief)."[29]

This southern reluctance to fund public relief societies and institutions, starting in the antebellum period, can be explained by the firm belief in racial separatism on the part of the white elite. Historian Timothy Lockley, who has written the history of public and private charities in the antebellum South, demonstrated that the white southern elite used to organize welfare distribution schemes only when they thought that poor Whites would benefit from it, because Whites "had a special status in society merely because of their skin color."[30] Before and after the Civil War, the white political elite resisted the development of public charity on the basis of social class only; race was the most important variable they took into consideration. These racial considerations added an additional political dimension to southern debates over whether black individuals should be granted their own asylum after the Civil War.

In 1877, the North Carolina General Assembly appointed a committee to find a site for the asylum for black patients. The newly selected site was just two miles west of Goldsboro. As early as 1874, the sum of $10,000 per year had already been allocated to the new institution, which was scheduled to be headed by the superintendent of the Insane Hospital of North Carolina (later renamed Dorothea Dix Hospital, after the famous campaigner for the opening of asylums throughout the country in the 1840s), which was located in Raleigh: "The general assembly of North Carolina do enact that the sum of ten thousand dollars per annum be and the same is hereby appropriated to the establishment . . . of a Branch Asylum for the Colored Insane and their support and treatment, subject nevertheless to the same control and general superintendance and regulations as the Asylum for the Insane at Raleigh."[31]

The opening of the Goldsboro asylum in 1880 changed admission rules for years to come. The other state asylum, the Insane Asylum of North Carolina at Raleigh, would no longer receive black patients, as it had, sporadically, since its opening in March 1856.[32] The Eastern North Carolina Insane Asylum in Goldsboro officially opened in 1880, more than five years after the state assembly voted to allocate funds to the institution. It is also worth noting that another institution opened three years after the Goldsboro facility, in the same state. The Western North Carolina Insane Asylum opened on March 29, 1883, in Morganton and received a budget surplus to host any white patient that the hospital in Raleigh could not receive. The budget surplus was voted by the same assembly in November 1874.

Comparing the admissions capacities for Blacks and Whites in the states of Virginia and North Carolina offers a striking example of racial inequalities in medical institutions at the end of the nineteenth century. In 1880, the state of Virginia had two asylums for Whites (in Williamsburg and in Staunton) and only one for Blacks (in Petersburg). At the same date, North Carolina also had two asylums for Whites (in Raleigh and in Morganton) and one for Blacks (in Goldsboro). No further state asylums for black patients were funded in these two states. Thus, from the 1880s until desegregation in the 1960s, the states of North Carolina and Virginia had a greater number of institutions and places for Whites, which would lead to problems of overpopulation in the institutions for Blacks.

In Louisiana, organizing the institutionalization of the black mentally ill population followed a different path, in part because of the French and Spanish heritage that shaped social and political institutions, and also because of race policies that had existed since the creation of the state in 1812.[33] Since 1843, the Société Française de Bienfaisance et d'Assistance Mutuelle de la Nouvelle Orléans, a French charity that offered assistance to the poorest in New Orleans, had offered care to its French-speaking members, black and white Creoles, against the payment of a subscription.[34] Catholic benevolent associations also played a large role among free people of color in the city who enjoyed high social status in New Orleans. The Société Catholique pour l'Instruction des Orphelins dans l'Indigence (Catholic Society for the Education of Destitute Orphans), the Colored Female Benevolent Society of Louisiana, and the Union Band Society all funded care for black patients in the antebellum period.[35] Prior to 1865, enslaved people were not allowed into state institutions, and only a few free people of color had been able to gain access to the Insane Asylum of Louisiana (later renamed the East Louisiana State Hospital) in Jackson, which opened in 1848, or to the New Orleans City Insane Asylum.[36]

In Louisiana, however, the treatment of black patients affected by mental disorders, whether they were enslaved or free men of color, was basic, principally because the Freedmen's Bureau set up after the Civil War failed to mobilize enough doctors or raise sufficient funds to come to the aid of this population in the southern states.[37] In a state like Louisiana, where part of the black population was free people of color and therefore had a unique status in the history of the southern United States, some black physicians practiced general medicine for the black population, though they remained very few in number. In 1870, only ten black doctors worked in New Orleans, giving a ratio of one black doctor for every 5,094 black inhabitants.[38] Historian John Blassingame reports a similar situation in 1880, when there were only thirteen black doctors, giving a ratio of one black doctor for every 4,434 black inhabitants.

Few of these doctors were university trained. Of the five black doctors listed by the Board of Health in Louisiana in 1882, only one, Louis Charles Roudanez, had obtained a medical degree from a university (Cornell). The black degreed doctors in Louisiana had not been through the medical school at the Medical College of Louisiana in New Orleans: Alexander Chaumette was a graduate of the University of Paris, while Isaiah Mullen and Thaddeus T. Walker had graduated from Meharry Medical College in Tennessee in 1883 and 1885, respectively. In the asylums and state hospitals in Louisiana, as well as in Virginia and North Carolina, the doctors and hospital staff, such as the nurses, remained primarily white personnel until the second half of the twentieth century (see figure 3).

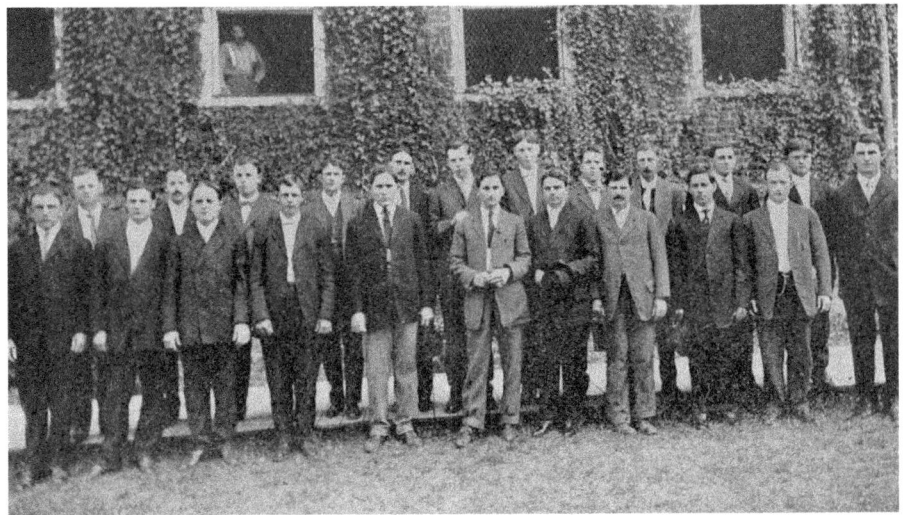

FIGURE 3. "Group of male attendants." From *Report of the Board of Administrators of the Louisiana Hospital for Insane ... Biennial Period Ending March 31st, 1910* (1910).

As a matter of fact, in North Carolina in the 1930s, Governor Clyde R. Hoey attempted to remedy the lack of appointments of black medical personnel in state institutions for Blacks, such as at the hospital at Goldsboro. In a letter dated September 23, 1938, and addressed to William A. Dees, attorney at law at Goldsboro and member of the board of directors of the state hospital, Hoey suggested that the board appoint black physicians in the very near future: "When we were talking the other day about the affairs of the State Hospital at Goldsboro, I intended to suggest to you that you discuss with the Board the question of designating some outstanding Negro doctors in the State as members of the Visiting Staff of Physicians for the Hospital." In his letter, Hoey anticipated that his proposal was unlikely to be approved by the board, whose members did not expect him to favor such an appointment: "Of course, I understand that you will select a white man as the doctor in charge, but I believe that it would be a very nice recognition to give to worthy Negro physicians to place one of them on the staff of visiting physicians for the Hospital."

To soften the blow, Hoey further argued that visiting physicians "are not paid anything, but they come to the Hospital at various times and perform services and operations and other things when called upon by the physician in charge." Hoey suggested that the board might support the appointment of a black physician under the condition that the job would be a temporary, unpaid position (and therefore precarious), under the leadership of the white staff. Mentioning that other institutions had arranged similar appointments, Hoey concluded his letter with the hope that the message would receive a positive response from the board: "If the Board of Directors think well of this and will indicate who they wish to designate as members of the visiting staff, I shall take pleasure in appointing them. This is the course pursued at both of the other institutions, and I shall be glad for you to call this to the attention of the Board at its next meeting."[39]

As could have been expected, Hoey's suggestion garnered only qualified support. On September 28, 1938, five days after penning his letter, Hoey received a response from William A. Dees, who, during a board meeting on the afternoon of September 27, had submitted the governor's request "relative to placing Negro physicians on the Staff of Visiting Physicians" at the State Hospital at Goldsboro: "The Board took the matter under consideration and called upon Dr. W. P. Holt, of Erwin, North Carolina, the only medical member of the Board since the resignation of Dr. John D. Robinson, to consider the suggestion together with the new Superintendent, Dr. F. L. Whelpley, who was appointed yesterday, and give the Board the benefit of their suggestions." The letter continued: "It was brought out in the discussion that there have been from time to time for quite a number of years suggestions and efforts from one source or another to connect up the Negro medical fraternity in the State with the operation and service in the State Hospital here. Though frequently the suggestions have looked plausible upon the face they have been determined as impracticable after careful consideration." The so-called impracticality, according to Dees, was due to several factors, which he penned methodically in an effort to make them appear plausible: "There seems to be some difficulty in the relationship between the White and Negro races and in the relationship perhaps especially between the White and Negro physicians which makes the operation of an enterprise by their joint participation impracticable. I do not think the situation in the State Hospital here is at all parallel, in this respect, to the situation existing in the Hospitals at Raleigh and Morganton." While assuring Hoey that "due consideration is being given to the matter by the Board," W. A. Dees ultimately rejected Hoey's proposal.[40]

A couple of years later, in 1940, the appointment of black physicians at the State Hospital at Goldsboro was once again the subject of debate, following the intervention of Charles Clinton Spaulding, the president of the North Carolina Mutual Life Insurance Company, a prominent black company located in Durham. Spaulding had a prolific career, as both a businessman and a leader supporting black civil rights. Aware that his own professional success would have a broader impact for future black business endeavors, Spaulding became active in politics and in 1935 helped establish the Durham Committee on Negro Affairs, serving as its first chairman. His political commitment to fostering opportunities for black professionals went well beyond the borders of the state. Indeed, he was appointed national chairman of the Urban League's Emergency Advisory Council from 1930 to 1939, and in this new capacity, he campaigned relentlessly to secure jobs for Blacks in the New Deal programs.[41]

On June 21, 1940, Spaulding wrote a letter to Governor Hoey to motivate him to appoint black officials in positions of leadership at the state hospital at Goldsboro, before the end of his term: "Before you leave office, I should like for you to have credit for doing just a few more outstanding things for the Negroes of North Carolina. I believe the persons heading our Negro colleges in North Carolina, the Morrison Training School for Negro Boys, and the Colored Orphanage at Oxford have proven their ability to successfully manage institutions operated for the race. In this connection we would like to see you appoint a Negro physician as Superintendent of the Goldsboro Insane Asylum for Negroes." Aware that this potential appointment would directly benefit the black community, Spaulding further stated, "Our state institutions which are operated for Negroes are the only place in the State wherein Negroes can demonstrate their ability to successfully lead others into worthwhile pursuits."[42]

Hoey sent his response to Spaulding on June 28, 1940: "I have your letter of June 21, 1940, and I note the suggestion which you make with reference to appointment of a Negro physician as the Superintendent of the Goldsboro Hospital for Negroes." Despite noting that "I fully appreciate your thought in this connection and I am anxious to have a Negro placed in charge of that institution just as rapidly as possible," Hoey was unconvinced by Spaulding's proposal and suggested that the potential appointment of a black superintendent would interfere with the work of the current superintendent, F. L. Whelpley: "The present Superintendent is doing such splendid work that I hesitate to interrupt at this time the splendid program for the improvement of this institution which is being put into effect. I may say to you that I just had a report from an outside inspector on this institution, and it ranks as one of the very best in the State. However, I shall bear in mind your suggestion and as opportunity offers, I think your plan should be put into effect."[43] According to Hoey, it was Whelpley who had caused the institution to rank as one of the best in the state, an achievement that reflected well on the governor's last term of office. Overall, the board's refusal to appoint black physicians in 1938 and Hoey's reluctance to challenge the status quo two years later further prove the persistence of a glass ceiling regarding the appointment of black physicians in asylums and hospitals treating black patients.

Unlike North Carolina and Virginia, the state of Louisiana did not open a single institution for black patients in the late nineteenth century. Unsurprisingly, just as in North Carolina, there were no black physicians appointed in state institutions until the middle of the twentieth century. However, Louisiana's unique political and social context regarding race relations at the end of the nineteenth century shaped the organization of institutions for the black mentally ill population. This was partly due to the mobilization of free people of color in New Orleans at the end of the Civil War to ensure the survival of their privileged status, and their access to public services and institutions on an equal footing with Whites. Their mobilization, which was successful, was organized to also avoid the exclusion of black patients from asylums and orphanages in New Orleans, especially when these institutions received funds from the city.[44] Mayor John T. Monroe testified in 1866 that "all persons temporarily insane are, without reference to race and color, admitted to the city insane asylum" in New Orleans, and when a correspondent from the *New York Herald* visited the asylum in July 1871, he found "white and black, old and young, pure and impure . . . all huddled together."[45]

Also in 1866, Mayor Monroe explained to Assistant Surgeon E. H. Harris of the Freedmen's Bureau that the Insane Asylum of Louisiana in Jackson was racially mixed: "I have never heard of any question arising on the part of the Superintendent of the State Asylum touching a distinction of races or color in the admission or non-admission of insane persons."[46] The asylum in Jackson, which was opened in 1848, was at the time the only other hospital that hosted mentally ill patients in Louisiana.

To alleviate overcrowding in the asylum located in Jackson, a second asylum was created. The Central Louisiana State Hospital, founded in 1902 in Pineville, also hosted black and white patients, organizing their living space into four separate sections according to sex and race.[47] The 1908 annual report to the governor showed that a "total of four hundred and seven patients" were hosted by the institution and that four departments had been created, for white males, white females, colored males, and colored females." This organization had been so set up because, according to the medical superintendent of the time, "the races and the sexes must, of course, be segregated."[48]

Admission to one or the other asylum in Louisiana was determined by parish of residence, not by race, unlike in Virginia and North Carolina, which had separate institutions for Blacks. The two asylums in Louisiana hosted Blacks as well as Whites, though in segregated wards. This is similar to historian Martin Summers's findings about St. Elizabeths Hospital in Washington, DC, which was the only federal psychiatric hospital to host both black and white patients, though there also existed the Canton Indian Insane Asylum, which operated from 1902 to 1934.[49] As Summers shows, the asylum staff at St. Elizabeths treated enslaved people who resided in the District of Columbia in the late 1850s; therefore, admission depended upon the residence of patients. As a federal institution, St. Elizabeths also hosted mentally ill soldiers and sailors from the 1850s onward.[50] Demographics throughout the nineteenth and early twentieth centuries in asylums and state hospitals in Louisiana, as well as in Virginia and North Carolina, bring to light a relative inequality in the number of places allocated to Whites and Blacks. In 1941, a total of 5,571 Whites were institutionalized by state institutions in Louisiana, compared to 3,237 black patients.[51] Since the beginning of the twentieth century, the hospitals in Louisiana had continued to see their white population increase, to the detriment of black patients.

Financing asylums for Blacks in Virginia and North Carolina, states that already had two asylums for Whites—the Eastern Lunatic Asylum in Williamsburg, Virginia, opened in 1773, and the Dorothea Dix Hospital in Raleigh, North Carolina, opened in 1856—was not self-evident. The public service mission in the case of black patients was reduced to the absolute minimum in the South, despite the efforts of black legislators. The decision to fund single-race institutions, however, foreshadowed by several years the doctrine of "separate but equal," which would be formalized nationwide with the *Plessy v. Ferguson* decision of 1896.[52]

In North Carolina, the opening of the asylum encountered strong resistance. Although the state was economically stable compared to the more southerly regions, states such as Alabama, Arkansas, Georgia, Louisiana, or

Mississippi, the issue of financing activities or institutions for Blacks was not a priority in the eyes of the lawmakers. An 1885 article published in the Wilmington, North Carolina, *Semi-Weekly Messenger* illustrates the reluctance to fund schools or asylums for black individuals. The paper opined that "while the north shuts out the kinky-heads and turns up its superior nose at the ill-fated scents, the south has for more than thirty years, in its poverty, and when struggling for bread, given a part of its earnings to the education of the negroes and to take care of their poor, their sick, their insane, their deaf and dumb." Yet, the paper continued, Blacks in the South had shown not one "particle of thanks and gratitude," despite the fact that "North Carolina has expended not less than 1,000,000 dollars on the education of negro children, since negro men began to vote against the men who employed them and fed their families to a great extent."[53]

This aggressive and polemical article reveals white southerners' resentment of northerners, or "Yankees," as well as of Blacks, who were seen as benefiting from public funds taken from the hands of Whites. Such arguments also existed in Virginia, where the Central Lunatic Asylum opened at a time when segregation was gradually becoming the standard for medical institutions in the South—despite the arguments put forward by the legislator Caesar Perkins, who fought against segregation in public institutions in Virginia. For an asylum for black patients to become a reality in Virginia, it was necessary to either build a new facility or create a segregated wing in an existing facility. Yet, equipping Virginia with a black institution that white taxpayers would help finance was not an idea that appealed to the majority of the population.

Martin Scott's letter to Robert F. Baldwin, mentioned earlier, evoked this reluctance to address the issue of black suffering in the South. The doctor explained that black patients should be sent to Massachusetts, a northern state where, according to him, former abolitionist Unionists would be happy to take care of their "protégés" rather than "inflict" on Virginia an additional cost—the rise of madness among black individuals being considered a collateral effect of the war. This reaction exemplified the dehumanization of the black population by the white elite, who refused to manage the social misery within their state and instead delegated their responsibilities to northerners.[54]

Similarly, one finds many newspaper reports of white reticence to cover expenses that would not benefit Whites, even more than thirty years after the opening of the Western Lunatic Asylum in 1870. On January 17, 1906, for instance, an article published in the Newport, Virginia, *Daily Press* reported that "the figures of the tax reports show that the negro pays a little less than 5 per cent of the money expended for the education of his child [while the] white man pays the other 95 per cent." The article added that "white people are taxed to care for the negro indigent and the negro insane in just the same proportion."[55]

Following this public debate, Captain Camm Patteson, a Democratic senator from Virginia, argued that public school funds and the funds of other public institutions, such as asylums, should be divided, so that each population, white and black, contributed only to the fund that concerned them. "It is a fair bill, and it proposes to keep separate the amounts paid by the negroes from that paid by the whites," explained the senator, pointing out that "the State of Virginia owes $73,000,000 of State debt, including the portion due by West Virginia, for which she is more or less responsible." He concluded, "The white citizens cannot go on at the rate we are going and pay for the education of the negroes of the State and pay the State debt."[56]

Patteson's arguments echoed the words of white conservatives in North Carolina and Virginia, who, since the Civil War (and throughout the twentieth century), had been protesting against the imposition of taxes, especially when the sums raised helped to fund public services for black individuals.[57] After the Reconstruction era, at the end of the nineteenth century, the voices against the financing of schools and asylums for black individuals sought to challenge black citizenship, and thereby to legitimize the exclusion of these new citizens from the public and political space, still thought to be the exclusive domain of whiteness. After the Civil War, the southern elite was fiercely opposed to taxation and intended to perpetuate a paternalistic model of public assistance, based on landowners' selective will to provide aid to their laborers, rather than a federal-based system of welfare. Paternalism was seen as a viable economic model because it allowed planters to find docile field workers at no extra cost; the white upper class could "tie black workers to the land in a world of free contracting, though not as firmly as the law had bound black workers under slavery, because coercion was no longer as viable and exit was an option."[58]

At the same time, planters promoted a form of assistance to their workers, which was based on racial separatism: the southern white elite decided to support poor Whites to the detriment of freedmen and freedwomen. They therefore satisfied their racial prejudice while promoting southern unity, which assured them the support of poor Whites. They only provided basic assistance to their black workers, "which they would forfeit if they were caught shirking." Therefore, the white elite used assistance and benevolence as a means to promote social control over their black workers and as a way to maintain the support of their white workers.

The same ideology was applied to the funding of distinct school systems in the southern states in the New South. The white elite, which controlled the local school boards in each state, were reluctant to allocate adequate funding for black schools in the South in the first half of the twentieth century. Consequently, "black Southern schools were decidedly inferior to those of whites" and "many blacks did not have access to high schools and had to travel long distances to attend elementary schools with poorly qualified teachers, primitive facilities and short term lengths."[59] More importantly, the improvements in black schools over the course of the twentieth century, at a time when black individuals were excluded from the southern political process, were due not so much to state funding as to private philanthropy by northern foundations such as the Rosenwald Fund, the Jeanes Fund, and the Slater Fund, and successful litigation by the NAACP in the 1930s and 1940s to demand equal funding. Public assistance and welfare for southern Blacks in multiple sectors, such as medicine and education, often came about only as the result of lengthy court battles and hard-won cases.

In North Carolina, the Goldsboro asylum was eventually opened in 1880. In the 1880s, the superintendent of the institution, J. D. Roberts, was pleased that legislators had agreed to fund this asylum for black individuals in his state, explaining in a paternalistic tone that "while there is a vast breach between the race and the tax paying portion of our citizens, socially, morally, politically, yet carp as the pseudo-philanthropist may, the old slave-owner is the negro's best friend, and has for him the most genuine pity in times of affliction." Roberts further commented that black individuals were "thrown on [their] own resources, with the cares of life and the support of [their] family, surrounded by temptations to indulge [their] passions, lusts, appetite etc., from which [they were] partially, if not wholly exempt in [their] slavery," thus reinforcing the argument that emancipation had caused higher levels of insanity than before in this specific population. To him, "it was no wonder that [their] mental balance gives way," since he saw his patients as being "improvident by nature, and not heeding the lessons of experience."[60]

Roberts thus pathologized the new social status that formerly enslaved people had gained after 1865—being freedmen and freedwomen after the Civil War and consequently enjoying new civil rights—declaring that insanity was being diagnosed in the black population in unprecedented numbers because their new experiences with freedom created new living conditions and looser social ties, which negatively influenced their mental condition. Roberts attributed predominantly white legislators' financial support of the asylum for black patients to their ardent paternalism and maintained that Blacks benefited more from such an institution than Whites, especially because they were imprudent "by nature" and less able, in socioeconomic terms, to take care of their own. Roberts's argument naturalized the socioeconomic differences between the two populations, to explain the need for the opening of these institutions.

The founding of separate asylums for Blacks in Virginia and North Carolina, and the opening of segregated wards in Louisiana, was but a short-term victory for the advocates of asylums in the South. Despite all the reluctance they expressed, southern Democrats could not forestall the construction of new institutions and segregated wings for Blacks, but they were able to limit their subsequent funding. From the 1870s onward, therefore, one can observe a progressive deterioration in the living conditions of black patients in southern public asylums.

In Louisiana, the treatment of black patients in the Jackson asylum after the Civil War was not without major dysfunctions, the most notable of which was massive overcrowding. Nevertheless, this did not give rise to a reassessment of the public endowment. The conditions of detention of the patients, both black and white, were no less deplorable in the municipal asylum in New Orleans. A reporter from the *New York Herald* wrote in 1871 that the patients of the institution "were dressed in all kinds of rags, some with shirts and some without, there they were talking, walking raving, sleeping or buried in their own sad, fearful reveries. . . . Glancing around in search of some appliances for the amusement and relaxation of the unhappy inmates, I found none. Not a book, not an occupation, not even a domino or a pack of cards." The journalist, depicting with horror the sinister atmosphere of the institution, also noted the presence of numerous instruments of discipline available to the physicians, should they wish to punish their recalcitrant patients, including "musketry, to fire on the Negroes in case they became refractory," which gives a clear indication of the attitudes that prevailed at this asylum.[61]

Poor conditions due to overcrowding likewise existed at the Jackson, Louisiana, asylum. Joseph Jones, a professor of chemistry and clinical medicine in the Medical Department of Tulane University, who also served as president of the Louisiana Board of Health from 1880 to 1883 and as president of the Louisiana State Medical Society in 1888, noted that the number of admissions increased sharply from 1870 to 1886, for both white and black patients, with white patients remaining in the majority. Jones noted that the living conditions of patients were deteriorating and that despite the increase in admissions, there was no increase in the public endowment of the institution. "Neglect, squandering of the public funds and suffering among the insane, characterized the years 1872 and 1873," wrote Jones, commenting that "over one-third of the inmates even in the cold weather of winter were barefoot and without shoes or stockings." Dr. L. A. Burgess, who was in charge of the institution in 1873, deplored that "absolutely nothing has been done to repair the decay and deterioration of the building, to remove the numberless inconveniences under which the institution labors, to introduce modern and labor-saving improvements, and to make the inmates comfortable, which is now far from being their condition," thus painting a dark portrait of his own institution.[62]

The neighboring institution, the Central Louisiana State Hospital in Pineville, founded in 1902, was overcrowded by 1912. It was built to accommodate 550 patients but was home to 639 in 1912, 685 in 1913, and 690 in 1914. Only a few years after the opening of the institution, white men and black women were sleeping on the covered porches of the asylum for lack of room in the dormitories (see figure 4).[63] In the 1920s and 1930s, black patients, unlike white patients, were locked in wire cages (see figure 5). Forty single rooms originally built in the black patients' wing had been converted into a ninety-bed dormitory (see figure 6). This overpopulation would last until the 1960s, when the institution was finally desegregated.

The disastrous situation of the Louisiana asylums mirrors the alarming living conditions of black patients in the Central Lunatic Asylum in Petersburg, where the asylum for black patients had faced a dire situation since its construction. From 1870 to 1915, there was an exponential increase in the number of patients.[64] Although the institution had received only seventy patients in 1869, with director Daniel Burr Conrad claiming that the asylum was "comfortably crowded," their number had reached 1,750 in 1915.[65] This sharp increase in the number of admissions triggered the lamentations of the hospital's

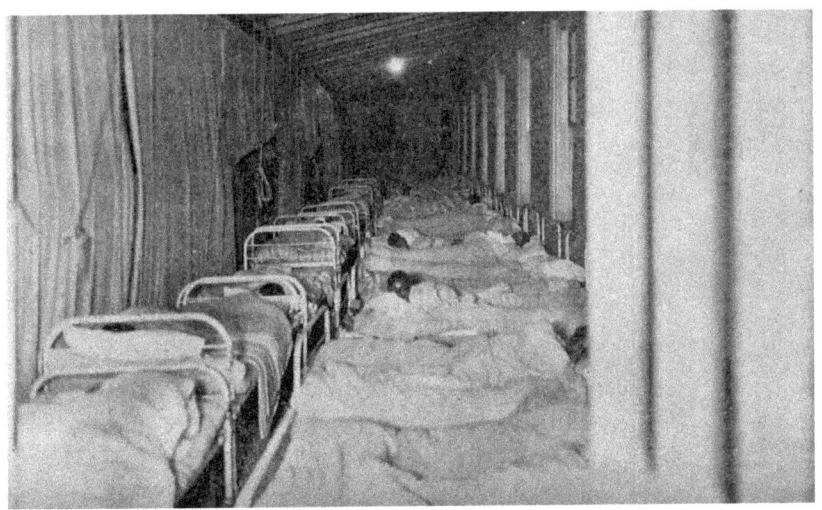

FIGURE 4. "Patients sleeping on Porches winter and summer—only canopy protection." From *Report of the Board of Administrators of the Central Louisiana State Hospital . . . Biennial Period Ending March 31st 1930* (1930).

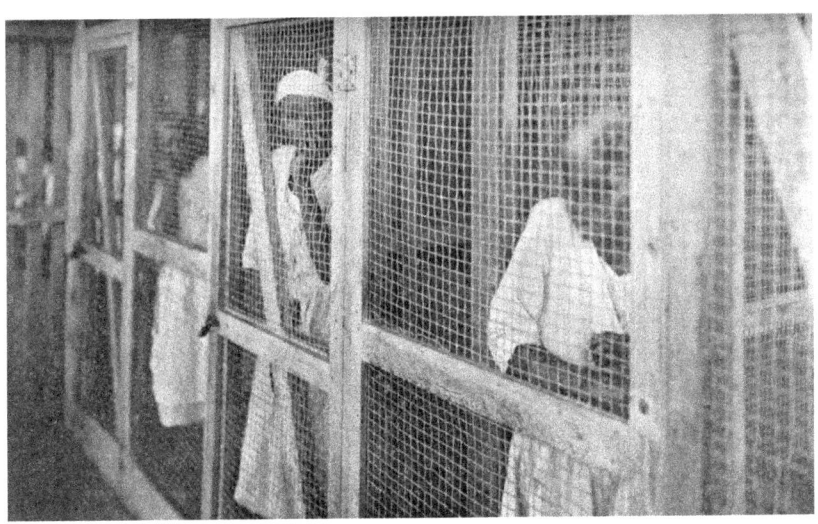

FIGURE 5. "Wire Pens and Cribs, before their removal." From *Report of the Board of Administrators of the Central Louisiana State Hospital . . . Biennial Period Ending March 31st 1930* (1930).

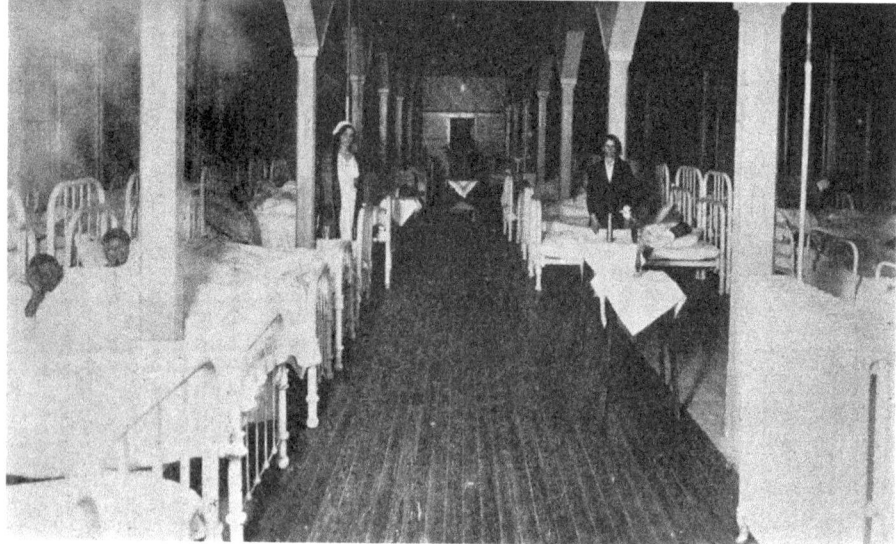

FIGURE 6. "Forty rooms constructed into Dormitories, 90-bed capacity."
From *Report of the Board of Administrators of the Central Louisiana State Hospital . . .*
Biennial Period Ending March 31st 1930 (1930).

successive directors, who year after year seized the opportunity offered by their annual reports to the governor of the state of Virginia to demand a budget increase. "There were . . . doubtless, quite a number of persons who were kept at home or not reported, because the hospital was so overcrowded it was difficult to get a patient in promptly, and, consequently, they had to be kept in jail," admitted William Drewry, superintendent of the Central State Hospital in 1921, admitting his frustration at not being able to conduct his mission in better conditions.[66]

Despite the increase in the number of patients, the budget of the asylum for black patients stagnated and was not up to that of other asylums for Whites in the same state. For example, in 1919, the annual operating budget allocated by the Virginia Legislature for the Central State Hospital stood at $294,097.17 for 1,763 patients (or $166.82 per person per year), while in the same year the budget allocated to the Eastern State Hospital, one of the white hospitals, was $156,452.78 for 775 patients (or $201.87 per person per year).[67] Parallel to this dire financial situation, which had resulted in overcrowding as early as the 1870s, the physicians introduced cruel punishments, such as mechanical restraints, as historian Wendy Gonaver has shown in discussing the Central Lunatic Asylum in Virginia.[68]

The decrease of public funding allocated to black hospitals may be attributed to the absence of those few black Republican legislators who previously had been elected to the Virginia House of Delegates since the second half of the 1860s and who fervently supported the funding of asylums for Blacks, despite lamenting their segregated nature. After the end of Reconstruction, in the late 1870s, the black delegates gradually lost their influence, and as the white Democrats regained control of the institutions, public budgets for black education and asylums were reduced. The lack of funding also reshaped these specific institutions, which took a more disciplinary turn—a development that black legislators in Virginia who had supported the opening of the Central State Hospital could not have foreseen.[69]

A similar situation with regard to an asylum for black patients can be found in the neighboring state of North Carolina. In one of the first annual reports published by the Eastern North Carolina Insane Asylum in Goldsboro in 1882, J. W. Vick, who was the president of the North Carolina Asylum Directors' Council, addressed himself directly to Thomas J. Jarvis, then governor of North Carolina, to ask for an advance on the amount donated by the state to ensure the smooth running of operations and the timely construction of dormitories. "Of the funds now in the hands of the treasurer of the last two years' appropriations, the sum of 200,000 or more, will be required in improvements of the hill upon which the Asylum buildings stand, and to prevent washes," explained Vick, insisting that since "the Board have decided that these improvements are necessary and cannot be longer delayed," the state's endowment should be paid without delay.[70]

Two years later, the financial situation of the Goldsboro asylum was still far from healthy, while the number of patients continued to grow year after year. In the 1884 annual report, Superintendent J. D. Roberts noted a dramatic increase in the numbers of the black mentally ill, which was up by a factor of 238 percent, if one compared the 1870 and 1880 census returns. These statistics worried Roberts, who foresaw an even larger influx of patients in future years. The institution had already reached its maximum quota of patients in 1884, only four years after its opening, and this did not bode well for the future.

However, Roberts chose to delay the construction of a new dormitory for patients, for reasons of personal convenience. Roberts explained, "It will be more disagreeable to the Superintendent's family, than living in the center building, as the noise, profanity, vulgarity, etc. can be better heard." Roberts continued by arguing that his family would suffer from living in close proximity to the black patients. "The lady members and the children of my family will be more exposed at the view, and to the remarks of the patients than at present." Furthermore, Roberts argued, his family needed some outdoor private space. "A private family needs a back yard: in this case, the only back yard available will be between the Asylum and the house, in full view and speaking distance (only 30 or 40 yards) of the windows of the male patients." Roberts concluded that, in his situation, "with a family of girl children to raise, this is, in my case, a very serious drawback to the location."

The construction of the dormitory near his own personal residence thus was not a viable solution for Roberts, who preferred to sacrifice the well-being of the patients to maintain the enjoyment of the private garden of his home, which was out of sight of patients. To convince the governor not to allocate the funds to his institution for the construction of the new building, Roberts argued that it would not be necessary to place the new dormitory too close to the other buildings of the asylum (although this would deprive patients of running water and gas heating), opining that this was "by no means essential, and can be dispensed with."[71] Roberts's argument was eventually supported by the other members of the council and by the governor of the state, to the detriment of the black patients, who were ever more numerous in the institution.

Two years later, in the 1886 report, Roberts pointed to new material malfunctions that affected the general living conditions of patients, saying that he regretted "to have to report that the heating apparatus is not working satisfactorily." Roberts advanced that "it may be that the engineers in charge of the heating have never understood its workings," thus accusing the employees of incompetence instead of signaling the malfunctions as the direct product of the financial disarray.[72] Such a description shows the negligence of administrators at the facility, only a few years after its creation.

By 1889, the issue of overcrowding in the North Carolina asylum remained unresolved, as again evidenced by the annual report to the governor. "The colored population of North Carolina is about one-third less than her white population, and yet to this date, we have accommodation for only about one-fourth as many colored as we have for white insane," said Roberts, seeing that the Goldsboro asylum was only one of four asylums in the state and that the others only welcomed white patients.[73] While the black population represented one-third of the state's population, according to Roberts (and verified by the 1880 census figures), it was far from benefiting from a third of the available hospital beds. As Roberts remarked, this showed the very unequal conditions in which Blacks and Whites lived in asylums in North Carolina.

This lack of care in the asylums also reflected the racial ideology of white southerners and the political economy in the former Confederate states in the 1870s and 1880s. The era from the 1880s to the 1900s saw the rise of the Jim Crow system, which compartmentalized public and private life racially in nearly every realm, from hospitals to schools; to sidewalks, housing, public transportation facilities, restaurants, swimming pools, and outdoor parks; to cemeteries, entertainment businesses such as theaters, and libraries.[74] Starting in the late 1870s, the white upper class enforced these restrictive state laws in an effort to promote white supremacy and to prohibit any form of social mobility for black citizens. These state laws legalizing racial discrimination were overturned only in 1964, by the U.S. Civil Rights Act, except for the laws pertaining to segregated schools, which had been dismantled in 1954 by the Supreme Court's decision in *Brown v. Board of Education.*[75]

Political rights and black enfranchisement were also limited by measures that aimed to restore the black codes, highly restrictive laws designed to limit the freedom of Blacks and ensure their availability as a cheap labor force soon after the Civil War.[76] After 1877, the southern states passed new state laws implementing poll taxes, literacy tests, and grandfather clauses (which allowed a man to vote only if his grandfather or father had voted prior to the ratification of the Fifteenth Amendment)—fraud and intimidation aimed at preventing black citizens from using their newly gained voting rights.[77]

These new state laws, which effectively banned black men from voting booths, were all passed gradually, starting in the 1870s. For example, the state of Alabama formalized disenfranchisement by constitutional revision at the state's constitutional convention in 1901, during which the notorious grandfather clause was debated, after it was passed in the states of Mississippi, South Carolina, and Louisiana.[78] Similarly, state legislatures in the South passed pieces of local legislation intended to disenfranchise black citizens after the short window from 1867 to 1877, during which black individuals gained new civil rights with the ratification of the Fourteenth and Fifteenth Amendments granting them citizenship and voting rights, respectively, in 1868 and 1870.

Before 1877 and the end of Reconstruction, black legislators made their entrance into state legislatures in states such as Louisiana and Arkansas, and sixteen black senators and representatives served in the U.S. Congress.[79]

The Jim Crow laws also signaled the violent return of white Democratic rule. The Reconstruction era saw the rise of the first Ku Klux Klan and of Klan-like groups in many southern cities and rural areas, starting as early as the 1860s.[80] Klansmen were responsible for creating a climate of terror; these extralegal white mobs perpetrated acts of violence for the purposes of social and racial control in their communities. Lynchings of black men were systematized and became ceremonial events during which white families gathered, celebrating white supremacy and glorifying violence over black civil rights.[81] As historian Harvey Young reveals, black bodies became trophies that the white audience members collected as souvenirs and relics after the lynchings, thus showing how these ghastly rituals participated in shaping a distinctive southern culture in which blackness was commoditized and dehumanized.[82] A recent study led by Equal Justice Initiative revealed that 4,084 racial terror lynchings took place in the South from 1877 to 1950.[83] Psychiatrists crafted their theories about black minds and proposed solutions to black mental illness in this specific political and social context of violence; the dire situation of negligence and abuse that was the everyday life of black patients in state asylums mirrored the day-to-day hardships that black citizens faced during the Jim Crow era.

It therefore comes as no surprise that this situation did not improve with time, in the early twentieth century. In 1900, a decade after J. D. Roberts's testimony about the dire financial situation of the hospital in Goldsboro, the Democratic newspaper *The Caucasian* published an article in which the disastrous financial situation of the Goldsboro asylum was discussed. A total of 239 black citizens who had been sent to the hospital could not be kept in the institution's walls, for financial reasons, and had returned either to their families or to the streets. The paper reported that physicians "call on the Governor State and judicial officers [*sic*], county boards of visitors, legislators, county officials and the press and on every good citizen to aid these unfortunate insane."[84] In 1923, the *Public Welfare Progress,* a monthly publication distributed by the North Carolina State Board of Charities, listed institutional advances in the treatment of mentally ill men and women in the state. The Goldsboro hospital was described as "very overcrowded" and "beyond its capacity," with 1,195 patients in an institution that could only house 1,085 patients.[85] While the Raleigh and Morganton asylums for white patients had an annual budget of $444,000 and $445,000 per year, respectively, the Goldsboro hospital operated on a budget of only $235,000 for the same number of patients.

Overcrowding was still prevalent in the early 1930s in Goldsboro. In 1929, the sheriff of Rockingham County, based in Reidsville, North Carolina, wrote a letter to the governor of North Carolina asking whether he could turn over to Goldsboro asylum a certain Leticia Harris, a black person who had no resources of her own and who had been found roaming the streets. The director of the hospital, W. C. Linville, answered him, explaining that he "wished that [his staff] could admit all of these patients but it is impossible to do so." Linville further lectured the sheriff about the quota of patients his county could send to his institution: "Your County is due, as her proportionate part of patients here, twenty-two patients, and you now have about thirty-eight more than your proportionate part in the hospital. I don't know what you can do with this patient unless you can keep her in your County Home, and we may have to, in the near future, send back to your county some that we now have." Linville also reassured the sheriff that his staff was "doing everything we can to handle the situation in the State," but that they were failing to further accommodate more patients in the asylum. "It is going to be necessary for your County and many others, to make arrangements to handle some of these patients at home," commented Linville.[86] It was indeed budgetary restrictions that obliged state asylum doctors for Blacks to send patients home, which attests to the poor material conditions of the hospital in which patients and staff evolved.

Yet Linville's concerns about the overpopulation of his hospital were voiced in the era of eugenics, when public officials showed deep concern about rapid population growth and great interest in the potentialities of selective breeding through theories of racial improvement. "Between the 1910s and the 1930s twenty-nine states [among them, North Carolina] enacted and put into practice laws permitting the involuntary sterilization of the 'feeble-minded,' as well as the mentally ill, the epileptic, and sometimes the criminal," as historian Katherine Castles reports, thus showing that discussions about the constant population rise in the state asylums were very much part of the national debate.[87]

In fact, North Carolina was one of the first states to make the leap and install a long-term eugenics program statewide. In 1929, the same year as Linville's correspondence with the sheriff of Rockingham County, the North Carolina assembly passed a law designed to provide for the sterilization of mentally defective and feeble-minded inmates of charitable and penal institutions. A couple of years later, in 1933, the North Carolina Eugenics Board was created. The board operated with the theories of racial improvement through selective breeding; sterilization was one of the methods adopted to eliminate poverty and mental defectiveness and to "reduce the size of a presumably genetically unfit and unproductive surplus population," thus following Francis Galton's nineteenth-century principles of eugenics.[88]

Born in England in 1822, Galton coined the term *eugenics* in the 1880s and posited that desirable human qualities were hereditary traits. To him, resilient civilizations are built on the merit of individuals. His theories quickly spread to Europe and then the United States, where they found a particular context of application in the Jim Crow South. From 1929 to 1975, the North Carolina Eugenics Board approved the sterilization of more than eight thousand people, the third-highest figure in the nation behind California and Virginia.[89] The vast majority of individuals sterilized were women who had been diagnosed as feeble-minded. Many of those sterilized were inmates of state mental institutions, such as the Goldsboro asylum directed by Linville.[90] Although sterilization was applied to large numbers of black inmates, most of those sterilized were white women.[91]

Sterilization in North Carolina, as in other southern states, targeted impoverished and mentally ill women because, according to the board administrators, they needed "protection" and "guidance all their lives," and were seen as unfit for motherhood.[92] Indeed, the North Carolina Eugenics Board operated according to the Malthusian theory that sought to prevent fast population growth within the lower social classes. In the nineteenth and early twentieth centuries, proponents of Malthusianism were seduced by the principles of eugenics, since they thought that humane birth selection and the elimination of the unfit was the only way to produce a better society. The concerns that Linville raised over the overcrowding of the Goldsboro asylum therefore echo this long-lasting obsession in North Carolina, throughout the twentieth century, with preventing rapid population growth among those classified as "unfit."

All in all, the deterioration of the hospitals for the black mentally ill populations of Virginia, North Carolina, and Louisiana in the nineteenth and early twentieth centuries stemmed from a broader southern political and economic context. The poor living conditions of black patients in southern institutions at the turn of the century highlights the building of a long-lasting unequal medical system, which in turn influenced the installment and reinforcement of a distinct southern political economy built on exploiting and commodifying blackness for the profit of white supremacy. Overcrowding in these state institutions mirrored the rise of Jim Crow laws, which legislated that freedmen and freedwomen as well as their descendants were second-class citizens in the southern states throughout the twentieth century. Indeed, the all-white medical staff at these new institutions believed that the new social status that enslaved people had gained after 1865 provoked high levels of insanity in the black population, which in turn was seen as the direct cause of potential drawbacks such as overcrowding, as more and more incoming black patients continued to flock the hospital gates.

Chapter 4 will address the theories and treatments established by white medical administrators and physicians who sought to discipline racialized bodies through strenuous manual labor. As we are about to see, the political economy of the New South permeated the hospital walls, as work was used as the chief—if not the sole—form of treatment to cure black bodies and black minds in these state institutions.

4

RACE AND MORAL TREATMENT
IN ASYLUMS AND HOSPITALS
IN THE SOUTH, 1870–1940

The bees work.
Their work is taken from them.
We are like the bees—
But it won't last
Forever.

—LANGSTON HUGHES, "Black Workers" (1933)

I n April 1889, Dr. Joseph Jones delivered a long-expected address to the
Louisiana State Medical Society for its eleventh annual session. Soberly
entitled "Diseases of the Nervous System," his speech provided an ex-
haustive report on the latest medical advances in Louisiana. To an audience
composed of the Louisiana medical elite, Jones gave an account of the classifications adopted by the professors of medicine at his university to classify and
treat patients in the surrounding hospitals. In his speech, he offered the latest
definition, then in vogue, of what constituted madness or "insanity," a curious
pathology "produced by defect or disease of the brain, and . . . synonymous
with mental disease, alienation, derangement, or aberration, madness, un-
soundness of mind," and which was understood to be due to hereditary, environmental, social, or even political causes.

It was about this last series of causes—the political—that Jones chose to
communicate. Detailing the cases of madness that he had encountered during
his practice at Charity Hospital and in the public asylums of the state (in particular, the asylum in Jackson), Jones dwelled particularly on "political excite-

ment," which he framed jointly with "religious excitement" and for which he had "treated a certain number of cases," both excitements being "congenital imperfections of the nervous system" that manifested themselves by "chronic alcoholism and masturbation." In his opinion, "political excitement and certain political and race changes, such as those wrought by the great American civil war of 1861–1865," constituted mental disorders, causing the patient to enter a state of madness that Jones described as "demoniacal."[1]

According to Jones, the Civil War produced political changes of such magnitude (emancipation) that the population directly concerned (freedmen and freedwomen in the South) became more susceptible to episodes of madness. Himself a Confederate veteran and an active and enthusiastic member of southern medical societies, Jones defended a medical and political apparatus based on white supremacy and anti-black violence in the post-emancipation period by producing naturalizing discourses on black freedom and mental illness. In the last part of his speech, Jones talked about the white southern men who fought against the abolition of slavery until the end of the war, stating that these soldiers had not been subjected to the trials of madness and their mental faculties had been kept intact. Four factors, he said, were responsible for this: "1. the consciousness in the justice of the cause for which their lives and fortunes were risked, 2. the brave and hardy nature of the southern people, 3. the physical development and perfection of the men and women of the Southern States, 4. the four years of incessant marching, entrenching and fighting which characterized the campaigns of the southern army during the struggle (1861–1865) inured the soldiers to hardship, hard work, frugal and scant meals, and educated their minds to face, without a murmur, disease, disaster and death."[2]

Jones hastened to conclude that the "heroic struggle tried the hearts of the entire male population of the Southern States in the fierce fires of battle and prepared them to struggle manfully with subsequent degradation resulting from defeat," constructing a theory that the Confederate soldiers' extraordinary demonstration of masculinity and virility exercised during the war would prevent the onset of madness among white Confederate soldiers. While Jones described black men as sinking into madness due to the heavy burden of their new political condition as freedmen, he theorized that the southern white men, loyal to their ideals of yesteryear, saw their mental state reinforced by defeat.

This double, parallel theorization, which aimed to emphasize the supposed rise of madness among black individuals through comparison with the mental and moral faculties of Whites, immediately raises the question of the political ideals held up by southern doctors. Analyzing the medical discourse on black pathological bodies, produced by physicians such as Jones, shows how doctors constructed racial otherness and defined racial differences as epidemiological while pathologizing political emancipation and naturalizing their black patients' capacity to work in a docile way.

This chapter will therefore focus on how southern physicians organized therapeutic treatments to cure black patients in the asylums, and how work was conceived as a curative instrument for formerly enslaved people. I offer here an analysis of the new pathologies and causes of madness that white physicians theorized specifically among the black population in segregated asylums in North Carolina, Virginia, South Carolina, and Louisiana, from the 1870s to the 1920s. I look at the circulation and use in southern medical spaces of local classification categories, such as "political excitement," to count and classify black patients, as well as the evolution of new taxonomies of madness, at a time (the 1890s and 1900s) when new classification standards were being adopted by the international community.

This chapter also examines the organization of distinct racialized work spaces specific to black patients, whose care was organized in relation to physical work, thus illustrating white physicians' efforts to view patient labor as a curative tool for returning freedmen and freedwomen to sanity by bringing them back to what was seen as their "natural" laboring condition of enslavement. The theories relating blackness to labor in state asylums offer a striking view of the naturalization of black bodies as well as indicating the rise of new medical theories linking power, white authority, and the treatment of madness among Blacks in the post-emancipation era. Work spaces were organized along racial and gender lines in segregated state asylums such as the Central Louisiana State Hospital in Pineville, where white women, black women, white men, and black men were assigned to different work tasks according to supposedly distinct epidemiologies. The chapter also deals with the visual representation of these work spaces in photographs that show the hospitals, both indoors and outdoors, as well as white and black patients performing different activities, ranging from leisure to manual labor. Consequently, the chapter will also show how historians of the New South can use visual archives to document the behavioral theories and treatments of black patients through labor. Finally, the end of the chapter takes a slight turn and relies on critical race theory and whiteness studies in an attempt to shift the focus away from white physicians. This last part will highlight the strategies of resistance that black patients put into practice when confronted with the exploitation of their labor force.

During the years 1860 to 1870, the categories used to classify the afflictions of black patients in asylums echoed those used for the white population. White physicians categorized insanity as "blatant mental decomposition," a form of "inflammation of the brain," or "headache." During the Civil War, these reported categories of illness were more often given as the causes of insanity or its symptoms rather than constituting diagnoses per se, irrespective of whether the sufferers were black or white.[3] However, nineteenth-century psychiatric nosology did not usually focus on race; instead, it was "a hierarchical and trait-based attempt to classify discrete entities," often described as "chaotic," by historians of psychiatry.[4]

Psychiatric classifications of illnesses were only standardized, and only gradually, under the influence of German psychiatrist Emil Kraepelin in the 1890s. Kraepelin is often celebrated as the father of psychiatric classification and of modern psychiatry. In the 1890s he proposed a model of classification that distinguished two forms of disease: manic-depressive disorders and dementia praecox.[5] These sets of diagnoses were grouped together according to specific symptoms and similar courses of deterioration. His classification was soon adopted internationally.

In the 1870s, however, physicians in Europe and in the United States still gave their full attention to what they described as the "causes of insanity." They believed that mental illness was a single disease that manifested itself in various forms, according to the unitary concept of psychosis. These causes were listed by physicians, in an effort to understand what led individuals to develop mental affliction. These lists could vary from one asylum to another, according to the local context.

For example, in 1872, the administrators of the Central Lunatic Asylum for Colored Insane in Virginia detailed that two patients had been interned because of a "change of life."[6] As historian Ann Clymer Bigelow explains, the category "change of life" appeared in asylums to qualify the transition between the white southerners' living conditions before and after the Civil War.[7] Here, the category is used in an asylum for black individuals to signify emancipation, which was understood as having led to more or less significant attacks of madness in the patients. A few years later, the 1877 report of the same institution noted that two male patients were interned on the grounds of "political excitement," while a woman was interned on the grounds of "sudden emancipation." Three other patients also were marked as affected by a change of life, which explained their hospitalization within the institution.[8] Though these six patients accounted for only 1 in 38 of the asylum population (a mere 2.6 percent), the very existence of these categories reveals that medical classifications engaged with political challenges.

A couple of years later, the 1882–1883 report listed, quite indiscriminately, the categories "change of life," "political excitement," "sudden emancipation," and "excessive study," the latter category qualifying black patients who had gone to school and learned to read and write. A total of thirteen patients were classified in these categories for that year.[9] In 1883–1884, four men were classified in the "political excitement" category, fourteen women in the "change of life" category, four men and two women in "sudden emancipation," and one man in "excessive study."[10] The figures for 1886–1887 were still on the increase (the number of patients admitted had quadrupled since 1872): six men were interned for "political excitement," seventeen for "change of life," five men and two women for "sudden emancipation," and three men for "excessive study." In 1889, asylum doctors classified eight men in the "political excitement" category, eighteen women in "change of life," five men and two women in "sudden emancipation," and three men and two women in "excessive study."[11]

In 1891, the categories "change of life" and "sudden emancipation" finally disappeared from the count, though "political excitement" was maintained, with twenty-nine new admissions (all men) so categorized, as was "excessive study," used to describe four men and two women.[12] A year later, the "political excitement" category again included twenty-nine patients, "excessive study" described four men and two women, and the category "emancipation" classified five men and two women.[13] In 1895, thirty men were classified in the "political excitement" category, five men and two women in "emancipation," with five men and two women in "excessive study."[14] The 1898 report, for the first time since 1877, did not contain the categories "political excitement," "emancipation," "excessive study" or "change of life" to qualify the cause of patients' madness.[15] Thus, over the period 1877 to 1895, these categories coexisted with others more commonly found in asylums in the United States and in Europe, such as "hereditary" madness or madness caused by religion, family trouble, a blow on the head, grief, alcohol, masturbation (for male patients), or love.

These classifications paralleled the rise of social Darwinism, which is seen fully in the naturalization of the social dynamics at work in the 1870s. As a matter of fact, the notion of "survival of the fittest" as applied to human populations predated Charles Darwin's writings and his famous *On the Origin of Species*, published in 1859 in London. In fact, the idea emerged as early as the 1790s, with Thomas Robert Malthus's *An Essay on the Principle of Population*. In his book, Malthus defined a doctrine of selection based on moral restraints. He argued for "preventive checks" to limit the birthrate of the lower social classes and reduce population growth, which, according to him, was a burden on economic cycles. Some sixty years later, Darwin popularized evolutionary theories for the animal and vegetable kingdoms, which he derived from Malthus's essay.[16] His theories were widely read and became extremely influential in late Victorian Britain, as well as in the United States during the Progressive Era.

The term "social Darwinism" does not properly define the influence of Darwin's writings on intellectual trajectories from the 1860s and 1870s onward. Instead, it reflects the bulk of social and political theories that invoked Darwin and his principle of natural selection. Philosopher Herbert Spencer was part of the first wave of essayists who coined the expression "survival of the fittest," in his *Principles of Biology* of 1864, and he became a strong proponent of social Darwinism.[17] This social and political philosophy therefore tied scientific theories to political and economic goals—the betterment of society through natural selection of individuals classified as the "fittest." The various labels used in asylums to classify supposed "causes of insanity" exemplify the rise of social Darwinism within these institutions, which hosted a majority of impoverished patients. These labels, which were based on social and political changes such as emancipation in 1865, parallel the incursion of scientific claims into the political arena, which was catalyzed by the doctrine of social Darwinism after the 1860s.

These categorizations, adopted and applied in Virginia over the period 1877 to 1895, also echo the theories that would be put forward by Joseph Jones during his conference in Louisiana in 1889, demonstrating that these categorizations circulated in the southern region. The use of these medical categories, moreover, echoes the politicized diseases already described by Samuel Cartwright some thirty years previously, though in a very different sociohistorical and political context.

The categories referring to the emancipation of enslaved people clearly indicate differential racial treatment by doctors after the Civil War. Indeed, during the same period, the asylum for Whites in Williamsburg, Virginia, did not present similar classifications. In 1890, the classifications reported were "excitement," "religious excitement," "masturbation," "child-birth," "excessive grievance," "domestic troubles," and others that were found in asylums for Blacks.[18] Thus, the presence of the mention of "political excitement" or "sudden emancipation" as causes of madness demonstrates a medicalization of deviance and political change applied to black populations now freed. While, as we saw in chapter 2, the controversy regarding the census figures of 1840 undoubtedly contributed to the invention of "madness" as a public problem during the antebellum period, this set of pathologies continued to be discussed in relation to the emancipation of black individuals long after the Civil War.

How then can we explain the presence and the upsurge of these forms of categorization, all referring to emancipation, in the asylum for black individuals in Virginia, more than thirty years after 1865? First, we can observe that the labels created by white southern doctors at the end of the American Civil War to categorize mental pathologies affecting black patients were marked by the political context in place and by the bitterness that white southerners harbored toward northerners because of the armed conflict that had destroyed their economic and political systems. As historian George M. Fredrickson points out in *The Black Image in the White Mind*, during Reconstruction, while federal troops were distributed over the territories of the former southern confederation, southerners harbored an intense "Negrophobia."[19] This fear of freed black individuals emerged in a context of intense political frustration for Whites and was not, strictly speaking, one of the products or remnants of the slavery system that had been in place before 1865; instead, this emerged only after the war.

The resentment that grew during Reconstruction would continue to animate white southerners well after 1877.[20] Southern Democratic journals such as the *Semi-Weekly Messenger* of Wilmington, North Carolina, spoke of "Negro domination" to qualify the Reconstruction era.[21] This social and political climate, without a doubt, helped to shape the face of mental pathologies developed by white doctors, who were involved in large numbers in local political life for the safeguarding of the southern way of life.

Furthermore, the diagnosis of "political" madness can also be understood in relation to the economic recession. As historian Eugene Genovese notes, the emancipation of black individuals came during a period of economic recession in the South. While Irish and Italian immigrants were seen as taking more and more jobs in the big cities of the ex-Confederate states, such as New Orleans or Charleston, free black individuals, unemployed in greater and greater numbers in the big cities of the South, were seen by Whites as a source of economic nuisance.[22] Many white southerners considered free black men and women during the Reconstruction era to be behaving in an "arrogant" manner. For example, historian Joseph G. Tregle Jr. relates that, for the white population in New Orleans, free Blacks were seen as dangerous to accost, since "many went armed with knives and pistols in flagrant defiance of all precautions of the Black code."[23] The differential diagnoses of madness thus did not so much show an epidemiological difference between Whites and Blacks in the South (as local southern doctors thought) as it reflected a change in socioeconomic relations and a fear felt by Whites of a reversal in the relations of social domination between the two populations.

From 1870 to 1890, many doctors used their influence to publicly express their misgivings about the political situation caused by the war and Reconstruction. These doctors, having displayed their southern patriotism with pride since the 1850s, closed ranks with the Democrats. After the Republican victory in the 1860 presidential election, William H. Holcombe, a doctor from Waterproof, Louisiana, published a pamphlet calling for the establishment of a southern nation separated from the North.[24] According to Holcombe, the interests of the South could not be defended with the Republican Party in power, since the party was antagonistic to the values of the South. Holcombe's attitude echoed the campaign that southern physicians had waged from 1840 to 1860 to ensure intellectual independence of the southern medical field from its northern counterpart and to justify the slave system by resorting to racialist medical theories and arguments that insisted on a natural proclivity for manual labor among Blacks compared to Whites.

As was demonstrated in chapter 1, the medical trajectory of Samuel Cartwright, one of the pioneer theorists of madness affecting enslaved people proves the existence of an interpersonal network linking the political and medical spheres in the antebellum South. A fervent anti-abolitionist, Cartwright was also the theoretician of drapetomania and dysaesthesia aethiopica, two diseases that pathologized enslaved people's micro-resistances to the political and social antebellum order on the plantation.

Cartwright was no stranger to the southern political field. He had cultivated many friendships among elected officials and statesmen and had private correspondence with Henry Clay, senator for the state of Kentucky and the architect of the Missouri Compromise of 1820, as well as with Mississippi governor John A. Quitman and with Jefferson Davis, who would become the president of the Confederate States during the Civil War. In these letters, Cartwright gave medical advice to his friends, disclosed his latest medical theories on black bodies, and discussed the future of the American nation, making no bones about the fact that he shared his correspondents' proslavery views in the context of rising sectionalist tensions between the South and the North.

However, Cartwright was not the only southern physician to link his medical expertise to southern politics. In the 1860s, shortly after the war, Joseph Jones became one of the editors of the *Southern Medical and Surgical Journal*, one of the southern medical journals published in Augusta, Georgia. The aim of the journal was to share southern medical discoveries as well as "observations of the recent disastrous revolution" that had affected the southern states, allowing doctors to assume a dual expertise, medical and political, at the same time.[25] The *Southern Medical and Surgical Journal* preceded the founding of professional societies such as the Southern Historical Society and journals such as the *Confederate States Medical and Surgical Journal*, which had been established after the Civil War, through which doctors from southern states could express their proslavery political sympathies and continue building a southern memory identity distinct from that of the North.[26]

Stanford Emerson Chaillé, a professor in the Medical Department of the University of Louisiana in New Orleans, had also participated in a heated debate published in the local press about the capacity of the freedpeople of 1865 and their descendants to take part in the local and state elections in 1870s. This debate fueled the idea that black individuals were, in essence, deviant citizens who were not able to exercise their right to vote and who terrorized white people on election day, notably by preventing them from voting for another candidate than their favorite, whether that candidate was Republican or black.

"As an American, dating back to a Huguenot's escape from La Rochelle, I am not yet prepared to believe, that this ineradicable conviction is destined to be supplanted by the permanent establishment of the political principle,—fatal to republicanism,—that *the bayonet ought to rule the ballot*," explained Chaillé in an 1875 article published in the *New Orleans Medical and Surgical Journal*, thus implying that black Republicans and their supporters would have used physical force to make their voices heard in the first elections open to black voters. A year later, Chaillé wrote again in the same medical journal to support the same argument, this time concerning the presidential elections of 1876.[27]

The medicalization of politics through the use of categories such as "political excitement" in asylums thus paralleled a broader phenomenon, which was the politicization of the medical field, as voiced in the public pronouncements of southern doctors who aimed to destabilize the new civil rights of black individuals. Furthermore, Chaillé's, Cartwright's, and Jones's medical trajectories illustrate sociologist Andrew Abbott's theory based on a "jurisdictional" approach to expertise in the context of the New South. In his well-known book from 1988, Abbott describes professions as interacting systems in which professionals constantly compete for jurisdiction over professional work. Abbott showed extensively how, starting in the nineteenth century and then in the twentieth century, individuals in the fields of psychiatry, neurology, clinical psychology, the clergy, and social work all competed against one another to provide expertise in the management of psychological and personal problems, and particularly of what American physicians saw as "general nervousness."[28] Southern medical practitioners in the New South sought to extend their expertise over their black patients' supposed inability to cope with emancipation, in an effort to establish their own academic reputations. In the process, they also aimed to win jurisdiction over political and social matters relating to civil rights and to establish themselves as political experts on the supposed negative impact of emancipation on southern lives.

Similarly, sociologist Gil Eyal's theory of "networks" of expertise could be applied to this specific context.[29] These nineteenth-century medical practitioners not only competed with other professionals for resources to establish their expertise over social and political matters—namely, the consequences of emancipation on the enslaved population. They also assembled their expertise with other professionals, such as southern journalists, essayists, and politicians writing on the same topics, and therefore participated in this broader network of expertise. Their aim was the production of renewed means of social and medical control over freedmen and freedwomen in the New South.

In the context of the rise of this distinct southern medical professionalism, which fully supported the southern political economy, the causes of madness attributed to black individuals in state institutions in the South were not unlike those attributed to pathologize women, another population thought as deviating from the norm. While men were seen as more easily affected by madness following exposure to alcohol or syphilis, women were seen as prone to attacks of madness after being pregnant and giving birth.[30] Other causes were thought to potentially affect both classes, such as marriage (married men and women being seen as more prone to madness), education level (when too high and causing increased arousal of the senses), or heredity.[31]

The political causes of madness applied to black populations in asylums drew from medical arguments that had circulated in other countries and had targeted populations that, like black patients in the United States, were marginalized and whose political rights were contested. The medical argument concerning freedmen and freedwomen, which at the end of the nineteenth century consisted of defining madness as the result of their freedom, drew inspiration from the allegations aimed at discrediting the political action of the Communards in Paris in the second half of the nineteenth century. In 1878, the conservative essayist Maxime Du Camp recounted the events of the Commune in *Les Convulsions de Paris*, employing the metaphor of madness for rhetorical effect: "The Commune was merciless, and it killed everything that seemed contrary to its madness . . . When the wheels of the vast machine are paralyzed or distorted by revolt, . . . the wind of revolutionary madness blows." The Commune was described as "a pathological case analogous to fire sickness, choreic epidemics," that spread "under the influence of overexcitement, deprivation, the license of manners, proclaimed and repeated aberrations, maintained and developed by the abuse of alcoholic beverages."[32]

Furthermore, the categorizations that were applied in the asylums for black individuals were also somewhat similar to the pathologies of the supposed "madness" of immigrants in the 1880s. Immigrants' ability to fit into the American nation and to follow Americanized social norms was a subject of debate. In addition to that, an 1882 federal law made madness a criterion for non-admission by immigration services.[33] In 1903, the law was extended to new immigrants who wished to enter the country and who had suffered from more than two crises of "madness" in their country prior to their arrival in the United States.

These successive laws had the effect of blocking the path of many immigrants, mostly Italians and Eastern Europeans. After the 1910s, new waves of immigration took thousands of immigrants from rural regions in Italy and Eastern Europe to the doors of Ellis Island in New York, which was the gateway between Europe and the United States until 1924. Italians and Poles made the transatlantic journey from Europe to New York with their families before establishing themselves in industrialized cities such as Chicago, Detroit, and New York, or their neighboring states, such as New Jersey, Ohio, and Minnesota. Often in their twenties and thirties, immigrants sought manual labor jobs in factories and often attempted to recreate in their new neighborhoods strong social and ethnic communities that resembled the close-knit structure of their rural villages in Europe.[34] In general, these people had moved to the United States at the turn of the twentieth century in an effort to seek better living conditions for themselves and their families, as had previous waves of Catholic Irish immigrants in the 1840s and 1850s, following the hardships created by episodes of famine in Ireland.[35]

A congressional report published tables that aimed to identify white patients who had been born abroad and were interned in asylums in the country (mainly from northern states, such as Massachusetts, New York, Pennsylvania, or Rhode Island, or from California), to show that the U.S. government still covered the medical costs of these new immigrants. The table showed that the population of white Americans born in the United States suffered from madness at much lower rates and were less often interned, proportionally, than their white counterparts born abroad. For Congress, the Irish, Germans, southern Italians, and Scandinavians were judged to be the populations most at risk of including many diseased individuals among their ranks.

Commentators at the time observed that the madness of immigrants developed after their arrival on American territory at Ellis Island, and not before their inspection; hence the high rate of sick people in asylums in the different states, the medical costs of which were paid for by American taxpayers. They were "not obviously insane while at Ellis Island but were then in the early stages of the disease, which became well developed in a few months," and they thus "became public charges . . . nine months" after landing.

A combination of causes was discussed in the report, ranging from racial trends to environmental trends. "The business of the alienist" was defined as tracing "the relation between the classification of the immigrant races and the probable causes that make some of them seem so much more liable to insanity than others." The nationalities were discussed and ranked according to their degree of primitivism: "It is generally held that the nationalities showing the least liability to insanity are also among the most primitive in point of education and standard of living," since "the mental equilibrium is more frequently upset in the instance of the highly organized nationalities; that is, they show less ability to withstand the shocks of a new environment, the pressure of unwanted economic conditions, etc., than the nationalities lower in the social scale."

American doctors in charge of the report explicitly discussed the two causes, environmental and hereditary. In the same document, which was published at the initiative of the federal government, they described madness as developing in proportion to the number of years immigrants have spent in the United States: "It is significant that insanity is apparently most prevalent in the nationalities who were among the earliest immigrants to this country and contributed the sturdiest of their people." Physicians explained these discrepancies by noting that the "conditions of American life are conducive to an increase in insanity."[36] Despite this apparent paradox, the less advanced races, from the point of view of the ideal of civilization that doctors imagined, were seen as the least affected by madness. Here we find reiterated the core of the medical argument developed in the 1840s that considered madness impossible among black and Native American populations on account of their lack of civilization.

Furthermore, the classifications produced by doctors in the Virginia asylums for the period 1877 to 1895 evolved concomitantly with the census statistics. Physicians referred to the federal statistics to show that the number of black citizens who had become mad in the South after emancipation continued to increase. According to Judson B. Andrews, the director of the Buffalo State Hospital in New York State, Blacks had been especially affected by what he described as a wave of madness since the 1870s, after emancipation. In an article in the *American Journal of Insanity* in 1887, he argued that their minds were too weak to face the complexities of freedom: "In the negro race the proportionate increase of insanity is far greater than in any other division of the population." Andrews explained that "from 1870 to 1880, there was an increase in the census of the colored race of 34.85 per cent, while for the same period there was an increase of 258 per cent of the insane." And he linked this "large multiplication" of cases of insanity to the "emancipation from slavery and the consequent changes in conditions and life." "The causes are briefly told: enlarged freedom, too often ending in license; excessive use of stimulants; excitement of the emotions, already unduly developed; the unaccustomed strife for means of subsistence; educational strain and poverty," commented Andrews, who aimed to pathologize the new behaviors of freedmen and freedwomen in the South, more than twenty years after the abolition of slavery.[37] Andrews linked the large increase in the number of black patients suffering from madness in the country to the fact that southern doctors advocated the opening of new medical institutions uniquely for Blacks from the 1870s onward.

Such a hypothesis of increase was shared in 1890 by the physician in charge of the asylum for Blacks in Goldsboro, who explained that "the late exodus of our colored population from this State [in the Great Migration] has not materially diminished the number of applicants for admission into this asylum." "It is very apparent to my mind that insanity is on the increase among the colored population, and I have no doubt that the responsibilities which freedom imposes, and extreme poverty, which is the heritage of many of this class, may be considered as potential factors for this state of things," he explained. He also added that "while it may be assumed as a fact that the negro can exist and be comfortable under less favorable circumstances than the white man, having a nervous organization less sensitive to his environments, yet it is true that he has less mental equipoise and may suffer mental alienation from causes and influences which would not affect a race mentally stronger."[38]

In North Carolina, the medical administrators from the Eastern North Carolina Insane Asylum at Goldsboro used an argument very similar to Andrews's. Lamenting the increase of their patient population, they attributed this demographic change to emancipation after 1865. To them, the migration of black southerners from southern states such as Virginia, North Carolina, Louisiana, and Alabama to the northern industrialized states—which became systemic from the 1890s until the 1940s and is often referred to as the first Great Migration—did not affect the numbers of admissions of black patients to the hospital. In fact, admissions were rising.[39] Despite the stark decrease in the number of black residents overall in the state of North Carolina, which was due to multiple factors—the necessity of seeking manual jobs in cities, the desire to escape segregation and obtain better living conditions—the number of black patients admitted within the hospital walls was on the increase, which they interpreted as a sign that black citizens were becoming afflicted by insanity at a much higher rate than before. The physicians therefore pointed to the moral and physical degeneration affecting black patients, which deeply worried them; they feared moral insurrection, which could in turn affect public order. The figures for black immigration were thus used to naturalize a well-rehearsed argument in the 1890s: that black citizens were unfit for the sophistication brought upon them by emancipation, as they were seen as mentally weaker than their white counterparts.

Thus were the arguments developed about the 1840 census (examined in chapter 2) revived more than forty years after their publication. Doctors again used census statistics to prove the increase in the number of mentally ill black patients in the South and to show that black individuals were more often subject to madness when free. Doctors such as Theodore Diller published an article in the *Pittsburgh Medical Review*, a newspaper in the North, about how "before the war of the Rebellion, insanity was very rarely found among the Negroes of the South." "Only when these ignorant, simple-minded, happy people became free and were compelled to work and manage for themselves and in their work, compete with others, has insanity appeared to any notable extent among them," Diller stated, whereas "under the old regime, care, anxiety, and perplexity troubled them not," because "peace of mind with happiness and contentment was their portion." Diller added that "the proportion of colored insane to colored population is fast approximating that of the white population, which in 1880, was one to five hundred." He continued, "With desires for alcohol, venery and emotional excitement unchecked; with childlike simplicity in the affairs of the world it is not strange to find this alarming increase of insanity among the colored people." Diller then used this statistical comparison to argue that black individuals suffered from their freedom, because of their so-called primitive mind-set.[40]

The argument that freedom was a cause of madness among black people had gained credibility during the era of Reconstruction, even in the northern states, more than thirty years after the original publication of the 1840 census statistics. In 1871, this argument gained weight in the *Weekly Louisianian*, a New Orleans newspaper, which published an article entitled "Statistics of Affliction" in which census data was cited to inform readers that freedmen and freedwomen suffered from insanity at much higher rates than southern Whites.[41] As we saw in chapter 2, during the 1890s, dementia in the black population was still discussed in connection with the recent acquisition of civil rights. For instance, J. Addison Hodges wrote about slavery in an effort to prove that since the Civil War, "the negro race is especially liable to certain forms of nervous diseases."[42] These white southern doctors claimed that, since 1865, Blacks had felt nostalgia for their formerly enslaved condition, because freedom had led them to face the worries of everyday life and had disturbed their minds to the point of making them mad. The expression of these feelings on the part of the enslaved was thought to be the imprint of the paternalistic relation uniting enslaved people to the enslavers, even long after the end of slavery.

Thus, putting patients to work to produce agricultural resources or products to be consumed in the hospitals was highly favored by white administrators, who thought to kill two birds with one stone—promoting docility while finding a solution to financial difficulties that were crippling the state institutions for black patients. From their opening, asylums reserved for black patients in Virginia, North Carolina, and Louisiana met with increasing financial difficulties, as we saw in chapter 3, and in fact institutions in the southern United States were generally much less wealthy and endowed than institutions in the North. Historian Gerald Grob notes, by way of comparison, that southern psychiatric hospitals in the 1870s and 1880s allocated on average $129 per patient per year, compared with $200 for institutions in the East and $167 per year for institutions in the West.[43]

During the preliminary discussions about the location of the Central Lunatic Asylum in Petersburg, Virginia, lawmakers defended the need for access to 250 acres of farmland so that "its cultivation insures ample employment to the patients" at a rate of sixty-four square feet per patient, whatever their physical or mental condition. The city of Petersburg was finally chosen for the establishment of the institution because of its proximity to rail and commercial networks, "as an economical measure in buying supplies, and where the surplus produce could be sold in a competitive market," rather than Howard's Grove, located half a mile south of the city of Richmond, where the asylum had been temporarily established.[44] The prospect of having patients work in the fields was therefore one of the parameters that dictated the location of the asylum.

The work provided by patients also appeared to be the most viable solution for fostering institutional self-sufficiency and reducing public expenditure, such as by growing fruit and vegetables for meals. The asylum was thus conceived as both a place of confinement for the mentally ill and as a place of work for the patients, requiring the majority of them to perform many hours of physical labor to repay their debt to the state for their care.

In this way, the long hours of forced black labor did not stop after the era of slavery; the extraction of forced work in asylums is blatant proof of the restoration of slavery practices in the New South after the Civil War. In Louisiana, physician Stanford Emerson Chaillé wrote about making black patients work in the Jackson asylum to offset the expenses of the institution. He argued that "those who are supported at the expense of the State are required (if it can be done without fear of injury) to do such light work as they can, from four to six hours each day; during the season of planting, the men are engaged in cultivating the various vegetables of this climate." He added that the physicians "also find considerable employment for another class during the winter season, in chopping cordwood." Putting the patients to work also served the material needs of the asylum, since, for instance, putting patients in charge of wood-cutting activities meant that administrators no longer had to buy some wood for the winter months: "As we keep up during most of the winter some twenty-five fires, it requires a large amount of wood for this purpose, all of which we get from the asylum lands."[45]

Chaillé's commentary shows that the asylum was thought of as both a place of confinement for the mentally ill population and a place to extract work from the patients, most of whom were required to perform many hours of manual labor. Chaillé also makes it clear that the long hours of forced black labor did not stop with the end of slavery; it still existed in the asylums for black patients after 1865. In fact, forced labor was organized through various systems of racialized coercion in the New South. For example, sharecropping functioned as a system of labor coercion that bonded black laborers to white landowners who rented out land in return for a share of the crops produced on the land. Sharecropping emerged in the years after the Civil War, when cheap labor was needed on the plantations where slavery had once existed and newly freed black laborers had no rights over the soil and needed work to support themselves and their families.[46] While sharecropping gave laborers relative autonomy and freed them from the gang labor system that predominated prior to the Civil War, it created a system in which sharecroppers put themselves in debt and had to pay off the landowner for the use of tools and other supplies. Overall, the sharecropping system recreated a form of financial, social, and racial control over black laborers and their families.

Debt peonage—also called debt slavery or debt servitude—was another way of coercing black laborers. Under this system, newly freed laborers and their descendants were forced to pay off a debt with work, while vagrancy laws compelled Blacks into labor contracts after the abolition of slavery in the southern states. These laws were not repealed by federal agencies or bodies such as the U.S. Supreme Court until the 1940s. This federal reluctance to suppress debt peonage was due to racial prejudice as well as to the upsurge of southern political influence after the election of President Wilson in 1912.[47]

Other forms of forced labor in the South after 1865 were specific to the carceral institutions. The convict lease system—through which the state leased prisoners to private contractors to provide a wide variety of manual labor—demonstrated the continuation of forced labor practices in the New South, well after the antebellum era. The convict lease system was implemented widely in the southern states and gained momentum until the 1940s. Historian Alex Lichtenstein has shown how, in the aftermath of the Civil War, the convict lease system served specific economic functions, as it fostered "the cutting edge of southern politics and economic development" and was even part of the Republican politicians' political platform, rather than that of the Redeemers, who overthrew Reconstruction.[48]

The convict lease system answered the high demand by railroad promoters for cheap manual labor to build new infrastructure following the end of the Civil War, while cementing the social control of freedmen through labor. However, convict leasing can be compared to a system of "neoslavery," as it functioned as a form of racial control, while at the same time being lucrative for the state.[49]

The convict lease system took different forms over the years. For instance, in a state like Mississippi, as prison historian David Oshinsky has revealed, black convicts worked at Parchman Farm (the Mississippi State Penitentiary), where living conditions were "worse than slavery."[50] Similarly, black felons who were convicted for petty theft were sometimes sentenced to chain gangs for several months—a brutal system in which prisoners were chained together to perform physically challenging work as a form of punishment. Historian Talitha LeFlouria found that chain gangs and convict leasing also brutalized black female convicts and that gender conventions did not protect them from performing physically challenging, monotonous tasks; in Georgia, female convicts worked from "sunup to sundown" and had gender-specific tasks, such as broom making.[51]

Therefore, at the end of the nineteenth century, forced labor in asylums was part of a broader political and social economy in which labor was used to rebuild what was thought to be the natural relation between white citizens and the marginalized black underclass. White southerners set up these strategies to reassert white supremacy in the South while creating a vulnerable black underclass and a workforce that continued to be exploited until the late 1950s. In contrast to the systems of forced labor implemented in carceral institutions, however, physicians such as Chaillé purported to use labor as a tool for therapeutic endeavors and as a pathway to curability and redemption. They naturalized the relations between labor, docility, and blackness as a way to secure the restoration of their black patients' health in the context of the New South.

Indeed, patients' work in the southern state hospitals of Louisiana, North Carolina, and Virginia had to do not only with financial costs but also with moral treatment. In the first decades of the nineteenth century, Western physicians believed in the moral therapy postulation that activities organized in the specifically designed setting of the asylum offered a potential cure to madness. The central tenets of moral therapy practiced in asylums supported the provision of a regular routine of leisure activities and useful means of occupation conducted in the restful and aesthetically pleasing environment of the asylum.[52] Not only did moral therapy provide improvements in the treatment offered within the physical environments of the asylum, but also these very provisions were seen as ultimately beneficial for the care and recovery of mentally ill patients. Moral therapy promoted a belief that everything in the patient's environment influenced their mental condition and that activities within that environment possessed therapeutic potential.

This method of moral therapy did not emerge only in the segregated South to treat black populations; it is to be found in the writings of the well-known French physician and precursor of psychiatry Philippe Pinel, particularly in his *Traité médico-philosophique sur l'aliénation mentale* (sometimes translated as *Medico-Philosophical Treatise on Mental Alienation*).[53] In his treatise, Pinel recommended "manual work that captures the attention [of the insane] and attaches them by the bait of a slight lucre" to promote calm in the establishment but also to restore serenity to the patient.[54] Pinel's methods were exported to the United States, where traces can be found in notebooks kept by southern physicians as early as the 1840s. Pinel's work was quoted by Joseph Jones of the Medical Department of the University of Louisiana in the 1860s and 1870s, attesting to the circulation of the notion of therapeutic work, implemented on this occasion for patients in Louisiana asylums without distinction of race.

The notion of therapeutic work and moral treatment, however, took a new turn in the South when it was applied to control and cure the black population of asylums. In the 1840s, John Galt, the superintendent of the Eastern Lunatic Asylum in Williamsburg, Virginia, mentioned the application of these therapeutic work practices for black patients especially, in the antebellum context. Galt revealed how black men and women classified as insane were required to make themselves useful for the maintenance of the asylum by working within the institution. According to Galt, this practice favored, on the one hand, their distance from white patients, and on the other, their healing.

"By reason of their aid in washing, the colored insane females are found useful to the Eastern Asylum, and on the whole may be considered a profitable addition: their ward is also somewhat of a sinecure to the servant having its attendance," explained Galt. The superintendent advised other asylum administrators who worked with black and white patients that the best policy was to "place no intermediate officer between the superintendent and matron of the institution and the patients; the contrary being the case in the Virginia asylum with respect to the white insane."

"It will possibly be found in most Southern institutions for the insane which shall adopt the plan of admitting persons of color, that the facility of assimilating lunatics of this class with the servants of the institution, will render their isolation from the white patients a very easy matter," elaborated Galt, who thought that white patients should be isolated from the black patients and the servants of the institution. "For by proper arrangements, most of the colored insane might be employed in assisting the servants of the establishment who had external duties to perform, and they would thus be scarcely in the wards at all during the day." Furthermore, "outdoor labor may be considered especially suitable to them, as corresponding to their usual mode of life when sane."[55]

For Galt, the inclusion of black patients in such an institution would make it possible for administrators to obtain a free labor force. Galt was especially concerned by the white patients' needs and their isolation from the black patients. Such practices would be legitimized by the therapeutic action that work bestowed upon black patients, most of them being enslaved and thus seen as used to working long hours in the fields. The doctor here presupposed that the natural condition of black men or women was to be enslaved; thus, their cure would be achieved through forced labor, to bring them back to their so-called natural state.

Galt's words marked the emergence, in the 1840s, of the argument proposing the naturalization of the relationship between black patients and work. Galt's theory of work as a curative tool for Blacks is anchored in a longer history of asylums as places for the moral rehabilitation of black bodies. The term *naturalization*, which qualifies Galt's rhetoric, is not necessarily an equivalent of *essentialism* here. Biological essentialism, especially in relation to race, posited fixity. In the nineteenth century, polygenists such as Louis Agassiz, Charles Cadwell, George Robins Gliddon, Samuel George Morton, and Josiah Clark Nott believed in distinct biological, racial "essences," because they claimed that different "races" (conceived by them as biological entities) had different origins and were therefore defined through heredity, in a rigid and deterministic way. For example, naturalist Josiah Clark Nott of Mobile, Alabama, went to great lengths to describe how black and white brains were different in shape, and he thus posited that enslaved people's so-called fixed physiological nature prevented them from developing levels of intelligence similar to Whites.

In the Old South, polygenists such as Nott also rejected evolutionary undertones. As historian Terence Keel explains, polygenists thought that "races did not develop successively from inferior primitive to complicated modern as was suggested by Lamarck or the British naturalist James C. Prichard." This view would be later challenged by the theories of Charles Darwin, who "discovered that change, not fixity, was the only constant force in the universe."[56] In opposition to this logic, the term *naturalization* refers to a positive process in movement. Physicians such as Galt thought they could cure enslaved people and restore their sanity by putting them to work, as work was thought to be their "natural" state.

The naturalization of the relationship between madness, blackness, and work was also taken up by other physicians in the South, a couple of years after Galt's original statements. Physician Samuel Cartwright's writings were mentioned in *De Bow's Review* in 1850 for his demonstration that black crime was indeed a disease, treatable through manual labor in state institutions. The author of the article cited "rascality" as an example of pathological deviations affecting Blacks and assumed that this pathology could be treated by a stay in "public prisons, penitentiaries, pauper houses, as well as hospitals."[57] The asylum was therefore thought of as the place of redemption, functioning as a space where black deviance could be transformed into more productive developments.

The naturalization of the relationship between work and the healing of mental pathologies among black patients gained a new impetus after the Civil War. Institutions in charge of crime, such as jails or prisons, and madness, such as asylums, were built in North Carolina after the Civil War because, prior to the war, "the slave owners had been to a great extent the disciplinarians of the people who make up a large proportion of the criminal class of the South, the Negroes." Therefore, according to the North Carolina statesmen, a new framework of discipline was now required.

A 1923 pamphlet about the history of state asylums in the country explained that the creation of asylums was a necessary evolution, since they were to control a population that used to be under the authority of an enslaver. The "plantation master" was described as the "lawfully constituted person to keep [the slaves] in order." After the abolition of slavery, the author explained, "with the freeing of the slaves hundreds of ignorant or more or less irresponsible persons were at liberty," and consequently, "the insane [who] were troublesome and often dangerous if left at large" had to be confined, as did "criminals for the protection of society."[58]

The pamphlet informs us that the myth of black patients' successful treatment through moral discipline and social control was still strong in the 1920s. Furthermore, it reveals that the myth of the naturalization of the interwoven relationship between work, blackness, and madness was part of the prevailing white political culture of nostalgia for the stability of antebellum plantation society, which became the epitome of southern political order after the 1860s. Southern nostalgia for slavery became even more intense after the 1890s, and it further escalated in the 1920s due to the gradual social diversification of blackness and the growth of the black middle class, which entailed the existence of black mobility in the ranks of landowners, businessmen, and political leaders.[59]

The motivation among members of the black middle class to educate themselves, along with the mobilization of black men and women for social equality, were met with disdain at best and violence at worst, in a context in which white southerners felt nostalgia for the Old South.[60] In North Carolina, the disenfranchisement of black citizens in the 1890s was mostly due to white supremacists' efforts to manipulate ideas of race and gender in order to politically disempower descendants of enslaved people, in a local attempt to restore the former social order. This southern political culture promoting antiblackness and nostalgia expanded in the early twentieth century and reached new territories. As historian Grace Elizabeth Hale notes, it even rose to the national level during the Roaring Twenties.[61]

For example, in the 1920s, the Ku Klux Klan gained credence in states outside the traditional South, such as California, Indiana, Maine, and Oregon, and transformed itself from its antiblack roots to focus on other minorities— namely, Jews, Catholics, and immigrants—whose presence on American soil supposedly threatened the "old" ways. Southern political culture based on nostalgia and supposed Anglo-Saxon roots became even more prevalent and permeable as it mixed with broader national discourses to give new definitions of race and belonging. Consequently, the framework of discipline set up by asylum administrators and physicians who used labor as a therapeutic treatment of their black patients in the 1920s fully participated in this well-established southern political culture.

In the state institutions, physicians relied on a specific activity to install a disciplinary environment for patients and to control patients' bodies and minds: physical work, also called therapeutic work. Work in the asylums thus appeared to be a necessity for the new social order and was motivated by the need to respond to the atomization of relations between Whites and Blacks during the Reconstruction era, which had been formerly dictated by the patriarchal slave system.

The control of bodies through physical labor, however, did not involve only institutionalization in asylums. Schools for black children, including those offering technical and agricultural training, became the great building site for developing the control of bodies and minds during the Reconstruction era.[62] Such was the case at the Hampton Institute, established in 1868 in Virginia under the leadership of the American Missionary Association. The aim of the Hampton Institute was to guarantee new freedmen and their children access to an agricultural and technical education, by providing the basics of agricultural knowledge. At the time, teachers saw black children as naturally fit to perform tasks in the fields rather than being capable of receiving an education in the arts and sciences. The *Southern Workman and Hampton School Record,* published by the school, provides information on the institution's educational program, which is entirely centered on agriculture.

In an 1899 speech at the Haines Normal and Industrial Institute in Augusta, Georgia, a black teacher, Hugh M. Browne, argued that just as one should not "talk English to a Frenchman and expect him to understand us," the teacher should adapt his speech to the audience of learners he was addressing (black children), and thus should take care not to overtax or exceed their intellectual abilities. Browne explained what he saw as the low level of black children's development, compared to that of Whites, by referring to so-called scientific advancements. While the "white race" is presented as "questioning Nature for centuries, and has grown powerful thereby in every particular, . . . the history of our [black] race is well-nigh destitute of such talks with Nature and our development is deficient to the extent of this destitution."

Though he was black himself, Browne declared that black individuals "have not yet reached the possibilities of the deftness of our hands and the capacities of our eyes and ears" and that "our brains have not yet felt the necessity for stimuli other than those furnished by these natural endowments." Browne continued his observations, arguing that the difference between white and black children could be explained by their education and socialization and was therefore not natural in itself: "The average white child of developed parents in this country possesses a wider actual acquaintance with the implements of this nineteenth-century civilization than the average educated colored man," since "they form a part of his everyday life from the cradle up."

"But our children when they come to you, come from homes where are found exceedingly few, if any, of these implements," explained Browne, who felt that the lives of black children were defined by "the plough, the pitchfork, the hoe, the rake, the saw, the axe, and possibly the hatchet." In Browne's opinion, black children must focus on mastering manual work in order to advance their civilization, rather than competing with Whites in areas where he saw them lagging behind, since "the development of a race is not a mushroom growth, but rather that of the century plant." He concluded, "We would better make haste to train our children properly for the fields now open to us—for that which we have—or we shall find ourselves neither in possession of others nor of these; even that which we have shall be taken away."[63]

The school was therefore thought of as the place both for learning discipline and for working, which was conceptualized as the most appropriate activity for young black students in the country. There is no doubt that the circulation of theories legitimizing the propensities and strengths of black individuals for manual labor at school facilitated the emergence of theories of work as the means to treat mental conditions in asylums in the nineteenth century.

In fact, work had been an integral part of the functioning of asylums for black patients from the 1840s to the 1870s. Daniel Burr Conrad, the first superintendent of the Central Lunatic Asylum in Virginia, mentioned with enthusiasm the curative virtues of work in relation to the supposed laborious "nature" of black patients and their former status as slaves: "From our experience during the past two years, work with the hands is regarded here, as elsewhere, as the most powerful hygienic and curative agents and influences which are classed under the general heading of 'moral treatment,' and we are inclined to think that this manual labor is the chief, if not the only, means of cure we possess for this class of our insane, coming as they all do from the totally uneducated former slave class."[64]

In his statement, Conrad made a clear link between moral treatment in the form of labor and the supposedly innate propensity among black men and black women to engage in arduous labor. In his view, manual labor would restore sanity to these formerly enslaved people, only a couple of years after the abolition of slavery. Thus, he naturalized black bodies by justifying the use of labor as therapeutic. The black body was thought to find peace and normality under the control of white medical power, which in turn sought to rationalize the physical and economic exploitation of this newly free labor force.

Work was also a way for doctors to compensate for the lack of leisure activities available to patients. In an 1886 report, J. D. Roberts described the monotony of the lives of black patients locked up in the Eastern North Carolina Insane Asylum in Goldsboro: "We have no amusement hall or chapel, both of which are very desirable in an institution of this character."

"Our patients beg and plead for the privilege of attending divine worship, but I have no way of gratifying them," lamented Roberts. "For the first two years of my service, I allowed selected cases of the best patients to attend church over in town and had the assurance of the pastors of the different colored churches that the deportment of our patients was all that could be desired." Roberts saw religious services as potential activities to occupy the minds and the spirits of his black patients. However, he explained that "the past three years this privilege has been denied them, under instructions from the Board." Roberts reported that he preferred to curtail all forms of enjoyment involving music and dancing, since "it excites others in the ward." He also argued that the long winters in the asylum were the most unpleasant time of the year for his patients. "In pleasant weather, when they can get outdoors, they do not suffer so much, but in long spells of bad weather, time must hang heavily on the hands, with nothing to break the monotony of their lives."[65] Isolated and socially excluded, the patients could only indulge in activities related to physical work on the asylum grounds. Work was the defining feature of the asylum, where the lives of the patients were regulated according to the possibilities for exploiting their physical force.

There were only minor evolutions in the organization of the Goldsboro asylum between its opening in 1880 and the 1930s, as can be seen from the archives of the journalist and essayist Nell Battle Lewis. In her diaries, Lewis recounted the routine activities of the patients in the 1920s, noting that patients woke up every day at 7:30 a.m., with no possibility of getting up sooner or later; had breakfast at 8:15 a.m.; took a hydrotherapy course from 9 a.m. to 10 a.m. three times a week, followed by a massage; and then took part in "occupational therapy" for the rest of the day, with breaks for lunch and dinner as well as a half-hour walk in the afternoon. According to Lewis, the work carried out included "weaving, basketry, bookbinding, sewing, knitting, leatherwork, drawing and painting, wood-carving and metal work for patients well enough to be trusted with tools." They were supervised by a "staff of eight thoroughly trained women in this field."[66]

Work in the asylum was also the cause of accidents and injuries, sometimes fatal to patients. The evidence of these accidents is to be found in the short reports written by the doctors of the institutions. In a report dated November 5, 1920, the Goldsboro Asylum Committee noted that patient Ward Cornelius "from Rowan County was reported as having lost an arm through accident, having, as it is supposed, stepped behind the guard to the shredding machine and getting the arm caught in the machinery." The accident was reported in the course of a paragraph, and the tone of the report indicates that this routine-sounding event would not hinder the subsequent operation of the institution.[67]

More than thirty years after the opening of the Virginia asylum, the therapeutic potential of manual work was still being praised by the doctors of the institution. In 1908, they voiced the same generalizations and justifications for manual work performed by patients in the fields of the establishment: "The regular, simple life, the hygienic conditions, the freedom from dissipation and excitements, steady and healthful employment, enforced self-restraint, the freedom from care and responsibility, the plain, wholesome, nourishing food, comfortable clothing, the open-air life upon the plantation, the kindly care and treatment when sick, in those days, all acted as preventive measures against mental break down in the negro."[68]

These few words, drafted by William Drewry, director of the hospital in 1908, left no doubt as to the nature of the therapeutic ideology put in practice by the institution. Black patients, to flourish anew, needed a simple and repetitive living environment based on the lifestyle of the Old South. This tall tale was kept alive by the medical authorities, who recreated, in a mimetic manner, the social order that had disappeared, and so sustained a nostalgia for the South. Thus, the export of the therapeutic model of work in the postslavery South took on a very special local hue; it was interpreted in the racialized and segregated context of the South, where naturalizing difference justified the segregation of bodies in public and private spaces—and, by extension, their inequality.

Although slavery did not necessarily precede capitalism, as recent scholarship suggests, the free agricultural work provided to the state by black patients offers a striking impression of déjà vu, since it reproduced the social order and the violence suffered by enslaved people in the era of slavery but in the post–Civil War era, in a capitalist economic system.[69] By controlling black patients, and above all by limiting the "flight" of workers, which resulted in the destruction of the southern economic market, the medicalization of work in the asylum ensured continuity between the figure of the enslaved person (constrained to work) and the figure of the worker (naturalized as a born worker), whose labor was now linked to his supposedly innate psychological character.[70]

Work therapy, however, was not organized the same way everywhere. It depended on the patient population treated, according to a complex racialized and gendered division of labor within the asylum. The 1872–1873 report on the Virginia asylum indicated that tasks relating to physical work on the farm, as well as in carpentry and shoemaking, were reserved for men, while women mended clothes, did the laundry, cleaned surfaces, including dorms and dining rooms, and knitted.[71] This system, developed at the Central Lunatic Asylum, was reproduced in other southern institutions and underwent local adaptations, depending, for example, on whether the hospital treated both black and white patients.

In his memoirs, James Lawrence Thompson, officiating at the South Carolina State Hospital, evoked the racial and gender hierarchy between white and black patients. Thompson indicated that "it was customary to employ as many of the patients as possible—those who were in condition to work—both male and female, white and colored." The physician recalled that while "white females would make beds, sweep the floors, sew, work in the kitchen and even sweep the yards, . . . the colored females would work on the wards in various ways and in the laundry."

"The colored males did most of the rough work, such as working on the farm, cutting wood and the like," since "the white males were somewhat handicapped in their work as it was not customary to have the white and colored males working together." Thompson further justified this functioning by saying that the facility "did not have land enough to have the white males work on the farm, hence they were confined to work mostly in cleaning up the yards and

moving trash from about the building."[72] These tasks were formulated according to tales of white fragility, while the hardest physical efforts were assigned
to black men as a way to strengthen the social control of black masculinity
within the hospital walls.

The arduousness of the tasks appears to have influenced assignments
according to the sex and the race of the patients. The male body, which was
theorized by physicians as indocile, was subjected to the hardest physical tasks,
in the fields, while the women were kept busy with daily domestic chores. This
economic exploitation of the black body is reminiscent of the convict lease
system in the South, but now with the psychiatric institution providing an arduous control of masculinity.[73]

Labor was also an opportunity to organize racialized and gendered spaces
associated with the treatment of bodies in North Carolina. Very early in the
founding stages of the asylum in Goldsboro, the doctors in charge of the institution envisaged the setting aside of recreational spaces necessary for the care
of patients. In 1884, J. D. Roberts, the director of the institution, described the
organization of recreational spaces intended to stimulate patients and enable
them to recover their health. In particular, Roberts proposed to create areas
where patients could practice gardening and stated that the gardens should be
maintained by the patients of the institution. Flower growing became a popular activity, which ultimately surprised Roberts. "When I placed them in the
wards I was fearful that the patients would break them up, but much to my
surprise, not a single flower has been injured, though the patients have had free
access to them for two months."[74]

In 1886, just a few years after the inauguration of the Goldsboro asylum, the
question again arose of allotting spaces to organize the work of patients. "Another need is for additional accommodation in the work department for the female patients. As now arranged, we have three rooms in the attic, inconvenient,
inaccessible, and entirely too small for the purpose—rooms that are needed for
another object. We encourage our patients to work if at all possible, as a means
of restoration in many cases, and others as a sedative; and I am sure we would
have better results if we had better facilities for employing our patients."[75]

In the 1890 report, director J. F. Miller wrote that black patients were the
main producers of work inside the walls of the asylum, especially the sewing.
"As it is our custom here, our sewing department not only does all the mend-
ing for our patients, but makes all the clothing for the females and nearly all

for the males, including bedding—blankets excepted. The employees in this department of hospital work have been very faithful in the discharge of their duties, and with the aid of our better class of female patients have largely contributed to the economy of our administration, and been of great mental benefit to the patients employed."[76] Women were given domestic work, according to a gendered model that associated women with the home and men with outdoor work.

Finally, it is interesting to compare the racialized and gendered labor in the state institutions that welcomed both black and white patients. A collection of photographs taken at the Central Louisiana State Hospital in Pineville and at the East Louisiana State Hospital at Jackson, Louisiana, further illustrates the highly racialized and gendered division of labor within these hospitals in the late 1920s and 1930s. Some of these photos show occupational therapy activities for white men and women conducted in a spacious garden, the patients being seated on chairs placed in a circle. In other images, they perform manual work such as sewing, in the case of women (figure 7), or assembling wooden chairs, in the case of the men.[77] At the Central Louisiana State Hospital, white patients worked in a sewing room that had been reserved for them since the 1920s. Although these photographs seem to have been staged, they provide ample information about differential routinized activities and work sessions organized for black and white patients within the hospital.

These documentary photographs, which for a long time have been passed over by historians of medicine, were published in the annual reports of the institutions and presented to the administration of the governor of each state to illustrate the institutions' proper functioning. Camaraderie and social interactions among the white patients may have provided encouragement, aid, and defense against the hospital's regimen and acts of mortification. These photographs further demonstrate how the medical staff and the photographer aimed to construct a public image for the hospital as an institution committed to the curative regimen of moral therapy, all while catering to the tastes, proclivities, and activities of white patients.

The annual reports of these institutions from the 1910s and 1930s also include photographs of black patients, who are shown performing different tasks, also labeled as "diversional occupation" (figures 8 and 9). Black men are depicted hard at work mowing the vast lawn or cultivating potatoes in the extensive agricultural fields surrounding the hospital, while black women iron

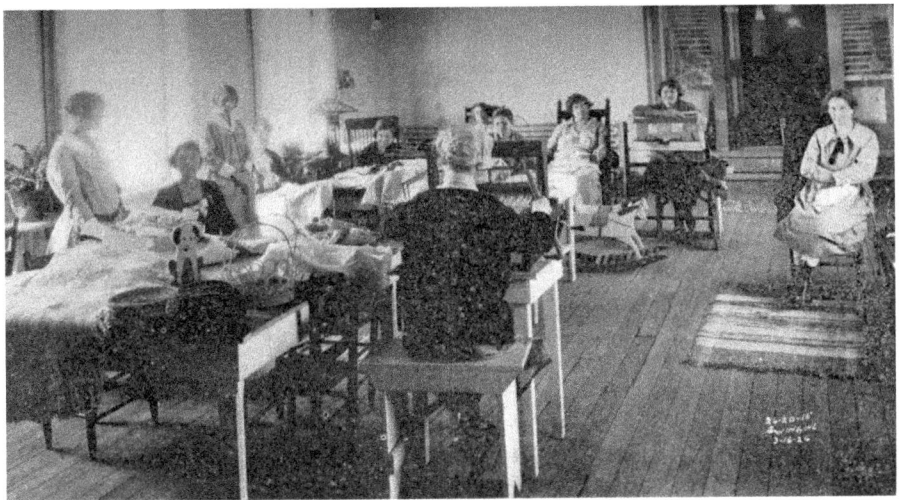

FIGURE 7. "Woman's occupational therapy room." From *Biennial Report of the Board of Administrators of the East Louisiana State Hospital ... 1924–1926* (1926).

clothes in a room in the main building, with no possibility of social interaction taking place among them.

These images contrast with photographs taken of enslaved people in the early nineteenth century, as shown by Matthew Fox-Amato's recent work. Fox-Amato states, "Through photography, some enslaved people nurtured a new, quiet habit of endurance and resistance on the eve of the Civil War." Enslaved people were themselves "photographic practitioners," who kept in their cabins "images of sold family members" and used these new representation techniques to offset "social and geographic instability." Furthermore, "as slaves lacked control over the mobility of their bodies and the categorical breakdown of these bodies into marketplace values, photography constituted a new mechanism to project and confirm full personhood and to endure the threat and actuality of constant separation."[78]

The photographs of black patients reproduced in hospital reports in the U.S. South convey a very different representation of black bodies. They seem to have been staged, since the patients are wearing neater clothes than usual. Since these photographs are reproduced in the reports of the institutions that were intended for the governor of the state, they present the hospital in its best light, as a site fostering patients' docility and their activities as effi-

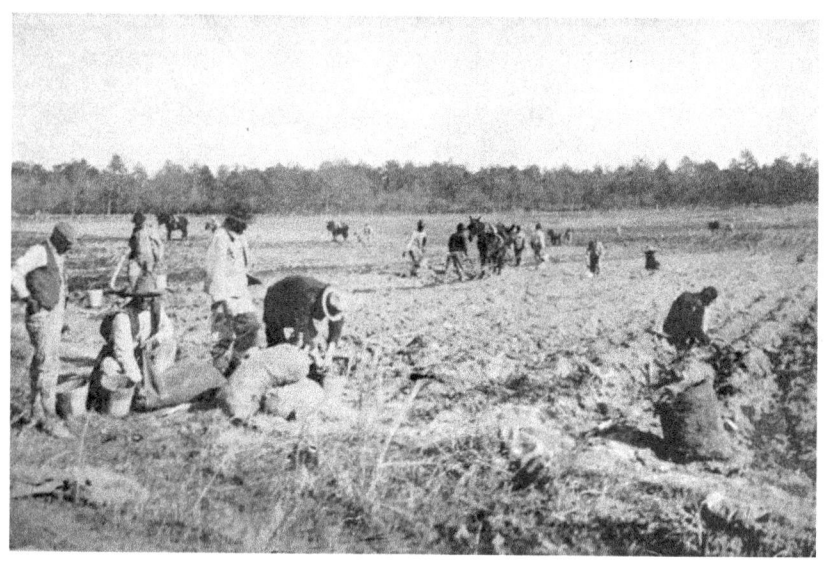

FIGURE 8. "Diversional occupation—patients cutting potatoes for planting."
From *Report of the Board of the Administrators of the Louisiana Hospital for Insane . . .*
Biennial Period Ending March 31st, 1916 (1916).

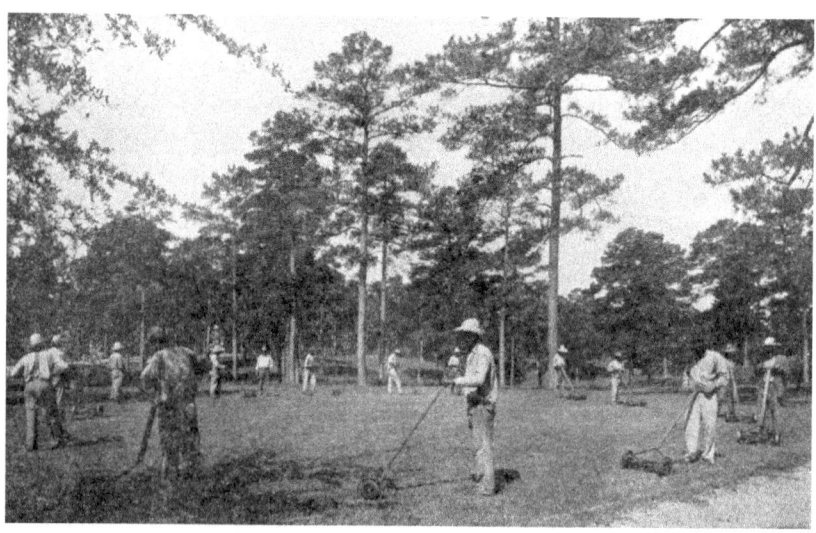

FIGURE 9. "Mowing Lawn." From *Annual Report of the Board of Administrators of the*
Central Louisiana State Hospital . . . Biennial Period Ending March 31st 1938 (1938).

cient laborers in the field. All in all, in these photographs we observe that black patients were required to do physically demanding manual work outdoors while white patients (men and women) work in indoor workshops and perform less exhausting domestic tasks, which reveals the differential treatments at stake for each given population.

The visual archives here underline that work was assigned to patients according to four categories: black male, black female, white male, and white female. These categories matched the increasing arduousness of the work. Black men were required to perform hard exterior work, such as tilling and mowing; black women were occupied with hard interior work, such as doing the laundry; while white men and women had leisurely indoor or outdoor occupations, such as light carpentry work, sewing, or hairdressing.

The visual archives that depict a gendered and racialized division of labor is further aligned with the patients' social origins and trajectories before their internment. A table published in the 1908 annual report of the Louisiana hospital lists the professional categories of white and black patients, women and men, across four columns.[79] Of the 102 farmers listed, only seven are white men, while seventy-one are black men and twenty-four are black women. The intermediate professions and qualified vocations are mainly held by white men; these are listed as "blacksmith, butcher, clerk, contractor (railroad), cotton buyer, journalist, pilot, mechanic, motorman, salesman, saloonkeeper, saw filer, veterinary surgeon." The white women are mostly housewives (forty-three, compared to twenty-two of the black women).

The work of black patients is designated by the (white) doctors of the hospital as leisure, even as black patients are photographed cultivating sugarcane, planting potatoes, or clearing a plot of land. The term "diversional occupation" is used in the caption for figure 8, as if the black patients were laboring for their personal pleasure. White women, for their part, benefit from a "beauty parlor" (figure 10), which was opened in 1931, while white men could take an outdoor gymnastics class. Black hobbies are synonymous with work, while Whites enjoy more relaxing and festive activities.

In general, the discourses of cure and recovery in such a "treatment" regimen were predicated upon the black patients' ability to work and upon their docility, whereas the discourse concerning white patients was centered around their capacity to espouse white ideals of domesticity, white vulnerability, and high social capital. Contrary to the systems of forced labor implemented in

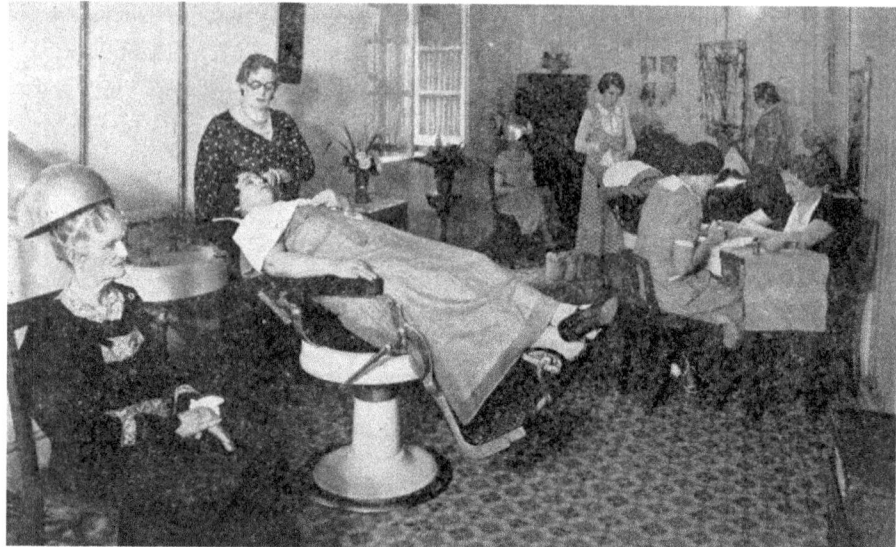

FIGURE 10. "Beauty Parlor." From *Annual Report of the Board of Administrators of the Central Louisiana State Hospital . . . Biennial Period Ending March 31, 1934* (1934).

carceral institutions, as shown in works by specialists of southern history and prisons such as Talitha LeFlouria and David Oshinsky, physicians used labor as a tool for therapeutic endeavors and as a pathway to curability and redemption. Overall, the medical staff constructed the public image of black patients at the Central Louisiana State Hospital in the 1930s in relation to former theories of labor, docility, and race that had started to be developed in southern hospitals all the way back in the 1870s. The superintendence effectively created two hospitals, each with its own distinctive ethos. On the one hand, it offered white patients a milieu that was therapeutic, comfortable, and based on the values of their social class. On the other hand, for black patients the hospital was primarily conceived as a workhouse in which manual labor was to be performed.

However, black patients were not necessarily passive and docile in the face of this arbitrary exploitation of their labor. From the early 1870s, voices of resistance emerged in the institution to protest the forced labor organized by white doctors, and these are reported indirectly in the institution's annual reports. Daniel Burr Conrad, the superintendent of the Central State Hospital at Petersburg, Virginia, recounted in 1872 that black patients' resistance to work emerged in his institution: "Some involuntary laborers . . . object to work, on the ground of its reducing them to their former slave state—'making them work without pay'; they say that 'if well enough to work, they are well enough to be discharged.'"[80] Patients' resistance exemplifies what philosopher Michel Foucault called "the insidious way in which madmen forcefully asked for the truth in relation to a psychiatric power which strove to impose its reality."[81] Here, it is not a "simulation of madness within madness," as Foucault puts it, but rather a revelation of the capacity for resistance by calling into question the arbitrary and coercive treatment put in place by the hospital staff.[82]

Such words are not isolated, either in the hospital for black individuals in Virginia or in other similar institutions located elsewhere. If the names and identities of these patients have often been erased from the registers (they are seldom named individually), these testimonies prove that black patients were aware of the contradiction between their status as patients and the work they were doing for free. Most of them (or their parents) had been subjected to slavery, and they recognized that their stolen labor was a vital contribution to their freedom, as work was a way to build their financial independence after 1865.[83]

For example, Abraham Tibbs, a black patient admitted to St. Elizabeths Hospital in Washington, DC, in 1910, was aware of the paradox of patients' work in state hospitals, which operated as punitive if not medical apparatuses: "The onliest time I got good sense is when I'm working for nothing, but when I ask for pay like you would, then I am out of my mind and insane."[84] To the violence of the white southern medical power, Tibbs opposes irony, and in so doing denaturalizes the power relationship that the doctor has striven to normalize. Against medical knowledge, he used his "subject knowledge," a form of knowledge that according to Foucault is deemed "non-conceptual . . . hierarchically inferior . . . below the level of knowledge or scientificity required," and he makes his voice subversive by bringing to light the unfair exploitation of his labor force in order to prove his right to freedom.[85]

This statement, which attests to the ability of black patients to resist their imposed labor, does not necessarily mean that white patients offered no resistance to the tasks presented to them. However, if resistance is not specific to black individuals, theirs is nonetheless more frequently reported in the archives than that of white patients, perhaps because it appeared to be more problematic in the eyes of physicians.

Evidence of resistance to forced labor, or to other treatments, can also be deduced from the institutions' annual reports of the number of patients who attempted to escape. J. D. Roberts, in his 1884 report on the Eastern North Carolina Insane Asylum, mentions that this phenomenon is due to the fact that "our patients have learned that the guards can be broken and several have escaped in that way." Roberts suggests that a solution to the problem would be to reduce surveillance and to put as many patients as possible to work, arguing that work is both curative and a disciplinary tool within the hospital walls. The flight of the patients also reveals that some of them were in good enough physical and psychological health to make up a plan and outsmart the guards. "Two of those escaped were so near well that no effort was made to retake them," Roberts explained, evoking the limitations of the institution, which was unable to prosecute patients or force them to return to the asylum.[86]

The 1920 annual report of the State Hospital at Goldsboro offers striking evidence of how patient escapes can be seen as individual acts of resistance to the rigid hospital apparatus in the early twentieth century: "It was reported by the Superintendent that George M. Irwin of Bruk county and Ed. Evans of Nash, patients, made their escape on the night of May 3rd, by bending the bars to their windows." George Irwin was later found "on the morning of the 4th . . . lying unconscious by the side of the railroad track about 10 miles from the Hospital." The hospital administrators reported that "he had fallen from the train, but just how the accident occurred was not definitely known."[87] These escapes demonstrate the ability of patients to free themselves from the medical yoke, despite the extensive medical and social control delimiting their daily activities, which was imposed by medical and hospital staff, all of whom were white.

Ultimately, the context of the opening of hospitals and asylums for Blacks in North Carolina, Virginia, and Louisiana reveals the existence of complex and contradictory debates. The evolution of the admissions statistics in the asylums was seen by the southern white medical profession as proof of the persistence of madness among black populations, which they understood to be produced by emancipation. The epidemiological reasons developed by white doctors to reject the costly construction of asylums in the South gave rise to the naturalization of the black body, alienating the individual and reducing their identity to that which was "innate," to a racial essence and a behavioral pattern that were theorized as fixed and unchangeable. In addition, southern physicians did not hesitate to create epidemiological categories that resonated with the recent political changes. Notions of "political excitement" or "change of life," which were directly applied to black patients in southern asylums after the 1870s and up to the 1900s, resonated with the broader history of the politicization of madness in other contexts in Europe, while showing an adaptation to the segregated way of life.

Furthermore, the racialist statistical arguments of the 1840s were put back on the agenda, in the context of the new social and political segregation that shaped the social fabric of the New South at the end of Reconstruction. A product of the new segregated era, the asylum is both its ambassador and its instrument, wearing the double face of black hopes and white social control, laying new chains at the feet of formerly enslaved people.

State institutions for black patients fell into a state of disrepair and overcrowding at the turn of the new century. They set themselves up as southern institutions in which a form of assiduous social control took hold. At the start of the Jim Crow segregationist era, they kept bodies separate, according to the precepts of white doctors that justified racial differentiation. Work surfaced as a tool for controlling bodies and minds—thus reproducing conditions of the slavery era—though it was given the appearance of a curative framework, precisely at the time when the madness of Blacks was understood as the corollary of their freedom.

Theories on freedom and insanity, however, were not voiced only in the South; they gained ground in the northern states, circulating in local newspapers in Detroit, Michigan, or through physicians in Buffalo, New York. It would therefore be wrong to assume that the pathologization of madness and race had only a southern focus. They certainly gained currency in southern physicians' reports and were applied in various southern state hospitals, but they also became part of a broader American medical apparatus targeting black bodies from the 1850s up to the 1920s. Furthermore, new theories legitimizing and naturalizing black individuals' strength and propensity for manual labor circulated in institutions such as schools for black children. In turn, such schools facilitated the emergence of moral treatment activities specifically designed for black patients, as the means to treat mental conditions in asylums in the nineteenth century.

Overall, the main concern in this chapter has been to show how the medical staff constructed the public image of black patients at the Central Louisiana State Hospital in relation to theories of labor, docility, and race developed in southern asylums at the end of the nineteenth century and the beginning of the twentieth. On the one hand, the superintendence offered white paying patients a milieu that was therapeutic, comfortable, and based on the values of their social class. On the other hand, for black patients the asylum was primarily conceived as a workhouse in which manual and even hard labor were to be performed.

Moral therapy offered remedial occupation and recreation, yet both options were not available to all patients. White patients were predominantly occupied with recreational activities—indoor games, theater, dance, excursions, and sporting activities—while the activities of black patients were mainly limited to manual labor, such as farm work and laundry. Black men were excluded from recreational facilities and were primarily occupied in providing manual labor for the asylum, assigned under the guise of occupational therapy. Black women were confined to the asylum buildings, where they performed domestic duties such as cooking, cleaning, washing, and ironing. Essentially, black patients were deployed as an unpaid labor force within the asylum.

The form of moral therapy that was offered to the white patients, on the other hand, included provision for the comforts and activities associated with their social class. The asylum did not strip white patients of the social and class privileges of their lives prior to institutionalization. Rather, one can argue that moral therapy recognized the importance of maintaining the prevailing norms associated with their social class. However, patients' testimonies and resistance provide evidence that compels us to reframe the official (photographic) image of the asylum and to see it as a visual fiction.

Work was thus the bridge or lever that allowed the care function to become a control function.[88] Initially conceived as a tool to liberate the mind, it was then used to subjugate fragile bodies to the legitimate violence of the state, of which the asylum institution was the ambassador. Rebellious voices nonetheless made themselves heard in the asylums, and they help sketch out the complex power game that existed between the representatives of medical power and their patients. There is no doubt that this subjugation of bodies and minds slowly and surely rekindled the flame of emancipation, echoing the lines of the poem "Black Workers" by Langston Hughes: "The bees work. / Their work is taken from them. / We are like the bees— / But it won't last / Forever."

5

THE FABRIC OF EPIDEMIOLOGICAL
OTHERNESS AND PATHOLOGICAL
BODIES, 1880–1940

In slavery I owns nothin' and never owns nothing. In freedom I's own
de home and raise de family. All dat cause me worryment and
in slavery I has no worryment. But I takes the freedom.

—MARGRETT NULLIN, in Eugene D. Genovese,
Roll, Jordan, Roll

The *Psychoanalytic Review* is the oldest continuously published psychoanalytic journal in the world, and the first printed in the English
language, which has assured it a broad readership. It was founded in
1913 by two psychiatrists, William Alanson White and Smith Ely Jelliffe, only
four years after Sigmund Freud's first visit to the United States. In the first volumes of the newly founded journal, John Lind, Mary O'Malley, and Arrah B.
Evarts, a group of psychiatrists from St. Elizabeths Hospital in Washington,
DC (where White also served as superintendent), published a wide range of
papers aiming to give the broader scientific community insight into the behavioral patterns of the black patients interned at their hospital. At the time,
St. Elizabeths was the only federal psychiatric hospital in the country, and since
its opening in 1855 it had been one of the first to accommodate mentally ill
black patients from the Washington, DC, area.

Published articles about black patients by doctors from St. Elizabeths are
of double interest today. First, they reveal the circulation of scientific knowledge, as the theories on black bodies and black brains published by the white
American psychiatrists at St. Elizabeths were deeply influenced by the read-

ings of European psychoanalysts. Second, they show the adaptation of broader psychoanalytic theory to a specific local context, namely, the segregated Jim Crow South. These articles highlight the way in which these American psycho-analysts, in the context of segregation, developed a politically charged medical framework along with theories to treat their black patients, in an attempt to "discipline and punish" black bodies—to quote Michel Foucault's well-known work about state institutions and madness.

I now turn to what I think is still an understudied topic in the field of the medical history of race: the development of psychoanalysis in Europe in con-nection to racialist theories in the U.S. South, and the history of local adap-tation of European theories to the segregated context of the 1880s to 1920s. Martin Summers's research has already highlighted the influence of Sigmund Freud on the practices employed to treat patients at St. Elizabeths, but Alfred Adler's psychoanalytical framework and its connection to southern racialist psychoanalysis has rarely been discussed in the historiography.[1] Throughout the chapter, I argue that the Americanization of psychoanalysis—which can be defined as the long-term process by which European psychoanalytic theories became introduced and then reused in different forms in the United States—has featured an often overlooked racial component.[2] The *Psychoanalytic Review,* launched just before World War I, did not restrict itself to publicizing Freud's analytic framework in the United States. It also popularized theories by Amer-ican physicians who treated black patients in the context of the New South and who sought to adapt European theories to their own moral, social, political, and economic context.

Most of these theories emerged and were applied specifically at St. Eliz-abeths Hospital, which stood as the primary social laboratory in which doc-tors such as William Alanson White, John Lind, Mary O'Malley, and Arrah B. Evarts could conduct various experiments and test the psychoanalytic frame-work on their black and white patients. Indeed, St. Elizabeths soon became one of the leading institutions where young physicians eager to know more about psychoanalysis and to incorporate these theories into their own prac-tices wanted to be.

William Alanson White became superintendent of St. Elizabeths in 1903, and his role was instrumental in disseminating Freudian theories in his insti-tution. On top of his administrative role, White pursued a publishing career in the *Psychoanalytic Review.* The journal had the specific goal of filling a gap in the medical literature published in the United States of the time. In a letter published in the first issue of the journal, renowned Swiss psychoanalyst Carl Jung praised the endeavors of Jeliffe and White for aiming at "the compilation of general psychological literature," which he described as an "ambitious enterprise . . . highly creditable to the liberal and progressive spirit of America."[3]

White's editorial activities were not limited to creating this new journal; he also authored or coauthored many books in the 1910s in order to share with the broader community the results of his latest theories based on psychoanalysis and the case files of his patients at St. Elizabeths.[4] One of his main interests was to develop specific psychoanalytic theories on mental development and race. In 1913, he translated *Dreams and Myths: A Study in Race Psychology,* a book authored by German psychoanalyst Karl Abraham, in an attempt to popularize Freudian theories on the psychic life of childhood and race psychology. Although Abraham's theories had to do with Jewishness, as he described at length "the wish dream of the chosen people and of the promised land," White's choice to translate this book into English demonstrates his motivation to make new theories on race and psychoanalysis available for broader use by American audiences.[5]

Looking at the specific articles by White and his colleagues at St. Elizabeths that were featured in the first year of the journal's existence is particularly relevant, as it offers a glimpse of the Americanization of psychoanalysis through its adaptation to the southern, racially segregated context—a relatively new process emerging in the 1910s and 1920s. Furthermore, these publications provide a direct insight into the theories and practices at St. Elizabeths hospital, as the articles often featured analyses of black patients' cases from that same institution. Consequently, this chapter can be seen as an extension of the study of the racialized theories and treatments that were implemented in southern institutions after the 1870s and were discussed in chapters 3 and 4.

I will first look closely at the ways in which southern physicians and psychiatrists categorized their black patients into distinct categories such as "mulattoes," "Africans," and "American Blacks" in their published research articles and medical reports. These classifications further prove that, from the 1880s until the 1920s, they attributed different symbolic meanings to populations that they theorized as epidemiologically distinct. First, the chapter examines the evolution of categorizations of black patients in the writings of physicians from Virginia and North Carolina from the 1880s to the 1900s, before the dissemination of psychoanalytic theories on American soil. It also examines the rise of new theories focusing on black bodies, culture, and biology after psychoanalysis became a new popular field in the United States in the 1910s, following the publication of the first volumes of the *Psychoanalytic Review* in 1913.

The advent of this new field of study in the early twentieth century reveals conflicts in the circulation of science, as the southern white physicians' local theories on black bodies and black brains were challenged by the readings of European psychoanalysts such as Sigmund Freud and Alfred Adler. Gradually, white physicians sought to adapt broader psychoanalytic theories to their own specific local context in the segregated Jim Crow South. Therefore, I will investigate the overlooked tensions between the process of standardization of science and local epidemiologies pertaining to the black population in the American context, and more especially in the U.S. South. In doing so, this chapter decenters the analysis from American to European history, showing the transnational influences of European physicians on American psychiatry.

Building on previous scholarship about the specific case of St. Elizabeths Hospital, this work also shows that the articles about race published in the *Psychoanalytic Review* over the short period of six years, between 1913 and 1919, mainly focused on three issues: the idea of primitivism embedded in black behaviors; the so-called sexual deviances of individuals categorized as black or mulatto, which physicians classified as symptoms of psychosis; and the act of passing as white as a proof of mental illness and deviance.[6] It also shows the transfers and circulations of this specific form of racialized medical knowledge in various southern states and American territories, such as Virginia, North Carolina, and Washington, DC, thus highlighting the spread of this racialist framework in the broader South.

In state institutions across the South, diagnostic classifications underwent a significant evolution at the end of the nineteenth century. In the South, and especially in Louisiana, mental disorders in 1906 to 1908 were classified as mania or melancholia and defined as "acute, chronic and recurrent," epilepsy, general paresis, idiocy, or even imbecility, including cases of nymphomania, paranoia, and dementia. Physicians applied categories to white males and white females, and to black males and black females, identified separately in the tables as "colored."[7] The race and gender population ratios were distributed proportionately to the number of patients in each category, except for the category of acute mania, where the recorded numbers of black men and women were twice as large as those of white men and women, despite their equal populations—a sign of a disproportion in this diagnosis for these two categories of patients.

At the Central Lunatic Asylum in Petersburg, Virginia, similar categories of diagnoses had been used to classify black patients since 1872. These included chronic mania, acute mania, nymphomania, melancholia, dementia, paresis, imbecile, acute madness, and delusional insanity, with no notable change in nomenclature until 1900, after which, subcategories such as dementia paretic, melancholia recurrent, melancholia stuporous were to be found. However, the categories of idiocy and nymphomania had disappeared from the classification tables by 1900. The category of dementia praecox (spelled *precox*) appeared in 1904, and more importance was given to the factor of heredity—a table was added to the 1906 annual report listing patients affected by hereditary madness.[8] The illnesses were called "psychosis" from 1909, rather than mere manifestations of "insanity," a sign of the specialization of medical vocabulary within these institutions.

The evolution of these classifications in Louisiana and Virginia is doubly revealing. First, the use of "dementia praecox" to describe black patients in the Virginia hospital from 1909 shows that the categorizations previously used had lost their aura by the 1900s. Second, the standardization of classifications followed the model developed by Emil Kraepelin in the 1890s, according to which diseases were no longer classified on moral grounds but as part of a continuum between manic-depressive disorders and dementia praecox, which would later be classed as schizophrenia.[9]

Southern psychiatry did not remain insensitive to the challenges of aligning treatment categories with those favored internationally. This led to an important transformation of medical practices, which followed, step by step, the publication of theories in peer-reviewed journals in Europe and in the United States. Prior to the intervention of Kraepelin's international classifications in the 1890s, diagnoses of madness were unstable categories and were described as all deriving from a single cause. As the international classifications of diagnoses (dementia praecox, mania, and so on) gained momentum, discussions based on a singular cause of madness lost their force of conviction. Madness was now understood to have several causes, including important hereditary biological roots.

The standardization of diagnoses also occurred at a time when American psychiatry began to follow different paths. While some doctors were moving toward an understanding of mental problems in biological or physiological terms, others were interested in neurology (the New York Neurological Society was founded in 1872, and the American Neurological Association in 1875). Still others, as early as the 1910s, were interested in Freudian theories of the human mind.[10] The standardization of diagnoses thus largely arose in response to this fragmentation of disciplinary fields, in an effort to medicalize hospitals and make them more scientific. Previously, the organization of hospitals had been the subject of criticism from neurologists, who criticized the directors of asylums for defining madness as an affliction determined by environmental causes. Neurologists saw state institutions as problematic and little useful; they considered that their directors behaved like autocrats or monarchs, reigning over their palaces with pills and handcuffs, without taking into account the latest scientific advances.[11] Thus, these developments—the specialization and empowerment of disciplines, the loss of interest in the unique cause of madness, and the advent of diagnoses—which significantly modified the content of the treatments and classifications adopted for black populations in institutions for the mentally ill, were part of a more general organizational movement.

However, southern physicians developed new classifications in relation to racial segregation. For instance, they used distinct racial categories to classify their patients, in an attempt to identify what they saw as various biological and natural traits relating to mental health. For example, in 1917, E. M. Green, then director of the Georgia State Sanitarium in Milledgeville, opined that Blacks were more affected by forms of psychosis such as dementia praecox than by depression, neuroses, or melancholia.[12] Similarly, in 1921, William Bevis at St. Elizabeths Hospital wrote that "sadness and depression have little part in [the Negro's] psychological make-up." Psychiatrists rarely diagnosed melancholia or neuroses in Blacks, which prompted psychiatrists Nolan D. C. Lewis and L. D. Hubbard to write in 1932 that there was a "low rate of depression among the negro as a race," without ever interrogating their own diagnostic bias.[13]

Physicians gradually diagnosed black patients with psychoses en masse from the 1920s to the 1930s, whereas they more often attributed to white men and women manic-depressive disorders, as doctors stereotypically viewed these diseases as appearing in patients with "more sophisticated" emotions.[14] Similarly, the diagnosis of dementia praecox had been associated with black populations in state hospitals because white doctors believed that "during its years of savagery, the race had learned no lessons in emotional control, and what they attained during their few generations of slavery left them unstable."[15]

Racial differences in diagnoses had long been produced, and then theorized as "natural," by white doctors in states such as North Carolina, starting in the 1880s. Throughout his career as a medical superintendent of the Eastern North Carolina Insane Asylum at Goldsboro, the only asylum for mentally ill black populations in North Carolina, J. D. Roberts isolated pathologies that he thought were more common among black or white patients. He explained, for example, that he had never seen a case of general paralysis in black individuals. Roberts conceded that "the predisposing cause for general paralysis" was "not definitely decided," yet he formulated hypotheses relating it to alcoholism, "excessive venery," "exposure to cold," as well as the "engagement in business affairs."

"If it is caused as some authorities hold by drink, it should exist to some extent at least in the colored race," explained Roberts. He concluded that "whatever its cause it cannot exist alike in both races or we would certainly see more of it in the colored man," since he could not seem to find in his own institution as many Blacks affected by this disease as white patients usually were.

However, general paralysis was not the only cause of insanity discussed by Roberts in the context of racial differentials. A few years later, in the 1889 report, he used the notion of emancipation to explain why so many black women in his institution were affected by madness. He and his colleagues claimed that "the number of female applicants had continued largely in excess of the male, and the experience of the past year strengthened the opinion expressed in a former report, as to the cause of the large increase of insanity among the females of the colored population." To them, "the heavy burden of responsibility which freedom had imposed upon this race is often thrown off by the men by abandoning their wives and children to an unequal contest for self-support, while they seek 'pastures new,'" thus linking bad marital relations to the more global context of emancipation after 1865.[16]

Roberts and his colleagues saw emancipation as negatively affecting the behavior of black women and the living conditions of black families, asserting that the new freedom that the men enjoyed led to them to abandon their wives and children. The physicians thus promulgated a medical judgment about the morals and ethics of freedmen in the post-1865 era; their new lifestyle was thought to cause insanity, which in the physicians' view partly explained why the asylum was receiving so many applications from black women in the 1880s.

Roberts and his colleagues dismissed the socioeconomic argument that could explain why black men sought work elsewhere. In doing so, they linked the madness of black women to emancipation, which, according to them, de-stabilized black families and led these individuals to their moral loss. Overall, therefore, white doctors were convinced that brain diseases affected Blacks and Whites differently, because of hereditary and biological causes embedded in the body and shaping race, and also because of the different social environ-ments in which individuals had evolved in the South—notably, under slavery for Blacks and freedom for Whites.

It is worth noting that medical theories that produced racial differences in the context of the 1880s, 1890s, and 1900s did not develop in a political vac-uum. They were deeply informed by the political context of the New South, whereby various journalists, political commentators, and white Democrats so easily labeled black individuals as impulsive, oversexed, undisciplined, credu-lous, superstitious, and savage.[17] Philosopher Angela Y. Davis has analyzed at length the black rapist myth in her book *Women, Race & Class* and has shown how young black men were commonly accused of rape in the South in the late nineteenth century and well into the twentieth century, following the emanci-pation of enslaved people and the gradual process of enfranchisement of black men during Reconstruction in the 1870s. She also discusses how sexual attacks on black women became a silenced "political weapon in the drive to thwart the movement for Black equality" as early as 1866, during the Memphis riots, when the "violence of mob murders was brutally complemented by the concerted attacks on Black women."[18]

As violence against black female bodies was made invisible in southern society, myths of white women's fragility and the danger of black men's lust erupted and permeated local news, widely shared cultural productions, and legal documentation such as court records.[19] As black struggles for freedom grew stronger in the 1890s, the wide local and national media circulation of depictions of Blacks as savage justified the lynching of numerous young black males by angry white mobs.[20]

Numerous routinized episodes of antiblack violence took place in the South, among them the 1898 Wilmington Massacre in North Carolina, which historian Laura F. Edwards states "became an affirmation of white supremacy not just in that one city, but in the South and in the nation as a whole." As Edwards relates, the riot came about in the postbellum context, and it "shook the antebellum household to its foundations, destabilizing the configuration of power it supported." In this context, black individuals became "the menacing, oversexed black male rapist and black female Jezebel, images that conveyed the extent to which Whites believed African Americans were incapable of self-governance."[21] In Wilmington, "physical discipline" and the coup d'état that followed the riot were therefore seen as "the only way to compel social responsibility" in a city where black men served as councilmen, magistrates, and police officers and where a black middle class thrived, composed of black doctors, lawyers, and educators.

After the coup, no black citizen served in public office in Wilmington until 1972. Moreover, no black citizen from North Carolina was elected to Congress until 1992, thus showing the long-lasting effect of this reign of terror in this specific southern state. This violent episode was no freak occurrence, however, as other riots followed—in East St. Louis, Illinois, in May and July 1917, and in Tulsa, Oklahoma, in May and June 1921. Both had been vibrant black neighborhoods at the turn of the century.

At the time, these outbursts of antiblack rage took place in a context that saw the rise of many cultural productions that were infused with growing antiblack sentiment and that even celebrated the southern political culture of lynchings. The nationally successful silent movie *Birth of a Nation,* directed by D. W. Griffith, chronicled and romanticized the rise of the Ku Klux Klan and culminated with scenes of Klansmen arresting Gus, a black character (portrayed by an actor in blackface makeup) who had pursued Flora, a white woman. It was the first American motion picture to be screened in the White House, in the presence of President Woodrow Wilson. Griffith unapologetically framed the Ku Klux Klan as moral saviors of the southern white order, while basing his story on popular myths about black male rapists, black primitivism, and white supremacy.

Similarly, in the 1890s and 1900s, numerous fictional works, such as Charles Carroll's *The Negro a Beast,* published in 1900, or Thomas Dixon's 1902 novel *The Leopard's Spots,* featured brute caricatures that portrayed black men as innately savage, animalistic, destructive, and potentially dangerous when in close contact with white populations.[22] These widely disseminated popular cultural productions fueled the racialist imagery that also informed antiblack policies and legislation in the South and medical theories on racial differences between black and white minds.

All in all, the psychiatrists' claims about innate primitivity circulated within a political culture that reinforced such ideas on the floor of Congress in the 1900s and 1910s. Cultural anthropologist and sociologist Lee D. Baker has demonstrated how, in public speeches, southern politicians such as South Carolina senator Benjamin Tillman, Alabama senator John T. Morgan, and congressmen from Mississippi referred to Blacks as natural-born savages and cannibals.[23] Tillman, a member of the Democratic Party who served as governor of South Carolina from 1890 to 1894, was known for his repeated defense of lynching and his efforts to ridicule and dehumanize black Americans.[24] These medical theories about primitivism and savageness therefore took part in the broader southern political agenda shaped by Tillman and others, which held white supremacy at its core and promoted it on the national scale at the turn of the century.

In this rigid political and social environment, modeled on theories about primitivism, antiblack politics, and the "one-drop rule" during the Jim Crow era, southern psychiatrists attempted to tackle one more specific problem: were biracial individuals (classified as "mulattoes" in the 1890s and 1900s) to be treated as white patients or as black patients? Indeed, the one-drop rule as a social, political, and moral principle of classification in the United States began to gain momentum in the nineteenth century, after the abolition of slavery, especially in the southern states, where the boundaries of black racial identity became defined by having one black ancestor—one drop of black blood through one's parents or even great-grandparents—regardless of phenotype or other social or cultural attributions.[25]

Following this principle of classification, southern psychiatrists were particularly preoccupied by the potential epidemiological differences among populations at the end of the nineteenth century. From 1900 to 1920, reports from the Central State Hospital in Virginia included the categories of mulatto and African, which physicians used to compare the distribution of diseases according to different phenotypes. This dual separation could also be found in peer-reviewed articles published in several journals about so-called mulatto populations, which, as historian Paul Schor reveals, was a term that was particularly in vogue in census classifications starting in the nineteenth century and up until the 1930s to classify multiracial individuals with mixed black or Native American ancestry.[26]

Doctors therefore understood an individual's race, seen as biological, as a significant datum along a colorist continuum that took into account the phenotype and the "mixed" genotype of individuals. Members of the medical profession particularly wished to theorize what they regarded as sexual deviance among mixed individuals whom they defined as mulatto. In an article published in *Alienist and Neurologist* in 1895, British physician Havelock Ellis hypothesized that individuals labeled as mulattoes were drawn to homosexuality, which at the time was regarded as a psychosis. Citing one of his colleagues, Ellis noted that "among the negro mulattoes of French Creole countries . . . homosexuality is very common. I know a lady of great beauty, . . . a stranger in Guadalupe and the mother of a family, who is obliged to stay away from the markets and certain shops because of the excessive admiration of mulatto women and negresses, and the impudent invitations which they dare to address to her."[27] Ellis highlighted medical beliefs about people he classified as such, as he considered them to be not only racially double but also pathological individuals with regard to their sexuality, which was assumed to be deviant.

Another article sheds light on the way in which individuals that physicians classified as mulattoes were treated as potential deviants in psychiatric institutions in the United States. Basing his theories on case experiments that he had worked on as an assistant physician at St. Elizabeths Hospital in Washington, DC, William Bevis wrote in 1921 that "mulattoes" were surely destined to become criminals, weak-minded, or both, because he thought the blood fusion to be particularly harmful to the mental balance of the subject, and that the white parent also represented a "defect," since they chose to associate with a black individual.[28] Bevis wrote, "If the original white parent were always even an average representative of his race, mentally and morally, the hereditary effect upon the more or less mulatto offspring would naturally be that of improvement of the traits and mentality of the colored race, but unfortunately the white man by whom this fusion of blood starts is most often feeble-minded, criminal, or both," thus stigmatizing the white parent for engaging in an interracial relationship.[29] This quote underlines how the medical and psychiatric apparatus actively participated in the regulation of the sexual norms and order at the time, by condemning and pathologizing interracial sexual relations, which were seen as immoral and unlawful in the southern states because they broke the taboo of racial mixing.

Similarly, the sexual behaviors of Blacks and the risk of sexual promiscuity with Whites occupied the minds of the psychoanalysts who published in the *Psychoanalytic Review* starting in the 1910s. Sexual deviance was a particularly common classification for Blacks in asylums in the early twentieth century, given that white social anxiety toward Blacks was often linked to a very high level of sexual anxiety, fueled by the fear of increasing promiscuity between the races. Arrah B. Evarts published an article in 1913 in the *Psychoanalytic Review* explaining that, unlike white patients, the black patient with dementia praecox was not remorseful about having satisfied his desires. Evarts wrote that the sexual instincts of black men differed from those of white men, since black men were "peculiarly unrestrained, and although they have learned much moderation, these desires are usually fully satisfied with no feeling of having done wrong." Evarts thus theorized that this lack of remorse on the part of Blacks accounted "for the fact that the ordinary sexual perversions are seen among praecox patients of the colored race much less frequently than among those of the white race."[30]

Evarts here naturalized the sexuality of her black patients as a case of deviance by installing a psychiatric biopower that matched the ambient sexual anxiety felt in the society of her time. Indeed, medical preoccupations such as Evarts's with the mulatto category and with black sexuality in general paralleled discourses from social and political commentators about sexual anxiety and the possibility of racial mixing between individuals classified as different "races." Historian Winthrop D. Jordan highlighted how "mulattophobia" became the norm in southern political circles in the nineteenth century, despite the fact that individuals classified as mulattoes had enjoyed "a special, higher status" in the earlier days of colonial America, during the 1730s, as the Anglo-dominated colony of South Carolina, for example, was more open about interracial sex than other territories.[31] This somewhat positive reading should, however, be nuanced, as the term "interracial sex" can be understood as a toned-down definition of the horrific sexual exploitation and rape of black women on plantation grounds in the eighteenth and nineteenth centuries, after the abolition of the slave trade, as historian Thelma Jennings reveals.[32]

Proofs of "mulattophobia" in political arenas could be found in hypodescent laws, which became part of the political arsenal of the southern states after the 1900s, as white Democrats regained political power after the 1870s and installed white supremacy in the former Confederate states. Tennessee adopted a one-drop statute in 1910, Texas and Arkansas in 1911, Mississippi in 1917, North Carolina in 1923, Virginia in 1924, and Alabama and Georgia in 1927.[33] These laws further limited the civil rights of individuals who could have passed as white in those states by assigning to their bloodline (and therefore to their descendants as well) the indelible stigma of blackness. While this classification of mulattoes versus individuals sometimes referred to as "full-blooded Africans" was not unique to the medical field (the census, for example, used such distinctions up to the 1930s), these new psychiatric theories delimiting so-called racial admixture certainly offered new justifications to southern political commentators and politicians who wished to tighten the social control and regulations regarding promiscuity of black and white residents in the South.[34]

In general, sexuality remained a highly debated subject among doctors in asylums and state institutions, with regard to black patients who were interned between the end of the nineteenth century and the beginning of the twentieth century, particularly in cases of sexually transmitted diseases such as syphilis among patients. The relationships between black men and black women were also scrutinized by physicians in North Carolina through the lens of sexuality. Diseases like syphilis and pellagra were very frequently diagnosed in southern asylums and hospitals in the early twentieth century, and they were quickly identified as common diagnoses touching black patients, leading to the creation of new measures in state institutions.[35]

W. C. Linville, the director of the Eastern North Carolina Insane Asylum at Goldsboro, wrote on October 10, 1929, to the state health officer of North Carolina, Chas. O'H. Laughinghouse, to explain that many cases of pellagra were listed within his asylum, causing forms of dementia and madness and leading to the deaths of patients. He declared that "out of sixty-four deaths which occurred in this hospital during the last three months, July, August, and September, twenty-seven of those deaths were due to pellagra, and that admissions of pellagra patients are very much on the increase." This increase put him and his staff "in a position not to be able to handle the insane that should be here." In reaction to the urgency of the situation, Linville soon announced that a committee would be appointed "to confer with the officials of similar institutions and the State Board of Health with a view of ascertaining, if possible, if there is any means by which the alarming increase of insanity, through preventable disease, can be stayed."[36]

Laughinghouse replied on October 11, 1929, saying that he welcomed this decision, and that he would arrange to have employed "a capable venereal disease specialist who will put on a program for the treatment of venereal disease in each and every one of [the] counties" in which the black patients lived. Laughinghouse also recommended a more generous allocation of funds "for the purpose of putting on an intensive educational campaign with relation to syphilis and pellagra."[37] Taken together, these different exchanges reveal that the sexuality of black patients in the Goldsboro asylum was gradually becoming a public problem, at the same time that doctors were scrutinizing the so-called harmful consequences of Blacks' sexuality.

However, southern physicians in the late nineteenth and early twentieth centuries did not reflect only on the mental development of individuals labeled "mulattoes" in relation to sexual deviance; they also looked at potential racial differences that could be located in the diagnostic grid and the mental dispositions that were thought to apply to Whites but not to Blacks. In 1891, A. H. Witmer, a physician who had worked at St. Elizabeths Hospital since 1876, before William Alanson White became superintendent in 1903, noted that black and white populations were evenly distributed on the diagnostic grid ranging from melancholia to dementia praecox, passing through different mania pathologies. In addition, Witmer created a distinction between the "full-blooded African Negroes," as he defined them, and the black Americans who had "mixed" genetic origins because of centuries of slavery having separated them from their land, and he found that, despite this distinction, his diagnostic grid was unable to differentiate them.[38]

Witmer's distinction shows that defining the exact influences of culture and biology on nosologies was at the heart of physicians' preoccupations. It also demonstrates the weight of racialized localism in medical practice in southern segregated institutions such as St. Elizabeths during the early 1890s. Furthermore, these new theories about sexuality and the supposed specifics of the psyche of mixed-race individuals followed the already established debates by southern physicians on race and epidemiology, which can be traced back to the 1880s.

In North Carolina in 1884, for instance, J. D. Roberts, superintendent of the Goldsboro asylum, discussed the so-called epidemiological differences in mental disorders among populations that he classified as racially distinct. Roberts argued that cases of suicide were not common among black patients, unlike their white counterparts, and he recalled that he had "seen so few suicidal propensities in the negro that I have advanced the opinion in a *Journal* article (N.C. Med. Journal, Nov. '83), that it was almost absent in the colored race."[39] In his article, Roberts noted that, in 1884, he had witnessed "the first attempt even at suicide that has occurred during my administration, and as [the patient] was almost white, I still hold to my original opinion that the colored man is not as prone to suicide as his white brother." Roberts further added that "this man would have easily passed for a white man in sections where he was unknown," thus making a link between phenotype, race, and the propensity for committing suicide.

Roberts's theories about suicide highlight the same concerns that Witmer held about biracial individuals in the 1890s. According to these men, the phenotype of their patients (whether lighter or darker) directly influenced their behaviors and actions. Only individuals that Roberts saw as his "almost white" patients (who were therefore still classified as black according to the standard one-drop rule in use at the time) could develop behavioral tendencies that were common to white patients, such as suicide.

Although overlooked in the historiography, Roberts's early theories on suicide, penned in the 1880s, also inform us of the ways in which psychiatrists of the 1880s, 1890s, and early twentieth century reflected upon notions of primitivism in relation to mixed-race individuals and black mental health. Roberts's quote can be linked to historian Martin Summers's brilliant observations about race, nosologies, and notions of primitivism in the 1930s.[40]

Indeed, Roberts's words were derived from his belief that black people had a childlike spirit and therefore were unlikely to consider committing the irreparable. Doctors such as Roberts spotted behaviors among black individuals that they described as infantile. According to him, for example, these patients would refuse food and resist the orders given by their doctors.[41] Summers reports a similar set of theories linking infantilism to blackness, which were developed some fifty years after Roberts's publication by Charles Prudhomme, a professor of psychiatry at Howard University. In 1938, Prudhomme suggested that his black patients were less affected by suicide because of multiple social factors, such as "their social oneness forced on them by the majority group, their still manifest urge to enjoy freedom, which is done only through living, and the consolation they derive from a religion that is so archaic." Similarly, Summers reports that B. J. F. Laubscher, who was a white South African psychiatrist at the Queenstown Mental Hospital, asserted that the "lack of civilization" of black individuals prevented them from even thinking of killing themselves, mainly because suicide was the product of the "stresses and strains" of modernity.[42]

Both Prudhomme and Laubscher, when writing about people of African descent, whether they resided in the United States or in Africa, linked phenotype to the notion of civilization. Since the 1840s, white physicians in the U.S. South had used this as a variable in studies on insanity, to measure the likelihood of individuals to be affected by madness, which as we saw in chapter 1 was theorized as the pathology of "modernity." Summers reports that these theories linking civilization to suicide were also developed by these psychiatrists because they "employed the language and concepts of psychoanalysis," which was a relatively recent field at the time.[43]

Interestingly, while Summers's article deals with these differential nosologies in the context of transnational exchanges between psychiatrists in the United States and colonial medical officials in Australia, Africa, and the Caribbean in the 1930s, after the development and dissemination of psychoanalysis in Europe and the United States, Roberts's theories predated the emergence of these new theories that focused on culture as well as biology.[44] Throughout the 1880s, Roberts was particularly accustomed to observing the alleged epidemiological differences between Whites and southern Blacks, which he linked to this same variable of "civilization." He published a pamphlet entitled "Insanity in the Colored Race," which appeared at the end of the 1884 Goldsboro asylum report to the governor. The same text had previously been published in the *North Carolina Medical Journal* in November 1883, demonstrating that Roberts had a sufficiently large audience, made up of both doctors and legislators. Roberts explained that "it is generally believed that the Negro, with other partially civilized or wholly uncivilized races, as for instance, the American Indian, is not liable to become insane as are the more civilized nations."[45] For Roberts, a lack of civilization was equivalent to infantile behavior.

Furthermore, psychiatric theories about blackness, primitivism, and mental deviance soon took another turn with the advent of Freudian psychoanalysis in the United States, starting in the late 1910s and 1920s. Indeed, psychoanalytical theories on childhood trauma, the interpretation of dreams, and theories on complexes and wish fulfillment were gradually adapted to the local southern racial context, even while they circulated on the international scene and, in particular, in the United States. The group of psychoanalysts from St. Elizabeths Hospital—Lind, O'Malley, Evarts, and Bevis—were instrumental in the circulation of racialist theses in the United States in the very first issues of *Psychoanalytic Review*.[46]

In their writings, these psychiatrists explored Freudian theories and spoke about the effect of the social environment and racial historical memory on the manifestation of psychosis in individuals. The writers were informed by early anthropological research that asserted that contemporary indigenous groups were still at the primary stages of human development compared to Western modernity. These theories developed side by side with other paradigms. While doctors explored Freudian theories, they continued to take into account the biomedical paradigm as well as environmental causes, in an era during which American psychiatry developed, from the 1920s onward, by following different branches.[47]

For example, Evarts, an assistant physician who worked in the women's wing at St. Elizabeths from 1912 to 1918, was particularly interested in linking previous existing theories about primitivism with neo-Freudian perspectives in treating black patients' cases. Using Freudian principles about the three levels of awareness that dictate human lives—the preconscious, conscious, and unconscious—she strove to analyze the beliefs that governed the daily lives of her black patients as signs that individuals, without knowing it, reproduced the primitive order of the advancement of their race. In the *Psychoanalytic Review* in 1916, she argued that "the influence of the race history permeates all thoughts and acts of the individual and yet he knows it not."[48] Evarts presupposed that the historical development of the "black race" as a whole (here seen as closer to the "barbarism" stage than the "white race") would have a direct influence on the behavior and development of the black individual. To support her thesis, Evarts took as an example the traces of voodoo practices that she found in her patients' behavior, considering these to be signs that marked the imprint of the historical substratum of the "black race" on the individual.

Her colleague John Lind, also a psychiatrist at St. Elizabeths, took up this vision of the black psyche as irremediably buried in a state of infantile barbarism, or "primitivism," as previously indicated by historian Martin Summers.[49] However, the links between this theorization of primitivism and medical experimentation on the black body and black mind has seldom been discussed in the historiography about psychoanalysis. In a 1913 *Psychoanalytic Review* article, during the first year of publication of the journal, Lind spoke of the links between infant psychology and the behavior of black patients. According to him, studies in psychoanalysis on Blacks in the United States could help forge a greater understanding of child psychology, especially since doctors had easier access to black bodies than to children to test their medical theories. "Although Freud has recommended the study of child psychology as a valuable aid to the understanding of abnormal adult psychology," he wrote, "it must be remembered that in his country there is no such race as we have here whose psychological processes are simple in character and so readily obtainable."[50]

"Perhaps to the American investigator, the negro might prove as valuable and more accessible than the child," Lind explained, seeing no ethical problem with experimenting on black patients to advance the study of child psychology. Lind formulated the hypothesis that since black populations did not reside in Vienna, Austria, where Freud was active in the 1910s, Freud was unaware of the possibilities offered by black psychological studies for the advancement of theories in child psychology.[51]

Lind's comment informs us that white American psychiatrists and psychoanalysts did not hesitate to recommend the medical exploitation of Blacks in order to advance medical science. Lind's remarks are not unrelated to the infamous medical experiments conducted fifteen years later at the Tuskegee Institute, on black patients who were mentally and socioeconomically vulnerable. Lind's comments also highlight a major paradox in the medical thought of the time: while black patients were understood to be epidemiologically different from white patients—black patients being placed in separate medical institutions and subjected to research that highlighted supposed biological differences between Whites and Blacks—these same patients were no longer thought to be radically different, from an epidemiological point of view, when the opportunity arose for doctors to conduct medical experiments on black bodies for the openly admitted purpose of advancing a so-called universalist science, which was thus applicable to all.[52] In other words, the racial exception advanced by doctors, which in their eyes justified segregation in the treatment of bodies, would no longer be necessary when profit was at stake, whether this profit was material or symbolic, such as for the advancement of science.

As a medical doctor at St. Elizabeths Hospital, which hosted both white and black patients, Lind contributed to numerous medical journals in the 1910s and 1920s, and he frequently acted as a medical expert in black psychology for his colleagues, advising them on diagnoses of black individuals in their own asylums. In a 1914 article, Lind developed a conception of biological race and attached great importance to the genetic admixture of the races, despite his use of psychoanalytic theories, which tended to leave aside biological mechanisms. Lind wrote that "[American psychiatrists] have to remember that we have in dealing with the Negro, especially the Negro with little or no white admixture, a somewhat primitive psychological type whose cultural levels overlook but slightly those of the savage," mentioning that "superstition still hovers with batlike wings over his emotions and casts shadows of fear about all incidents differing from his daily routine."

Psychoanalysts like Lind, despite their interest in the influence of the social, cultural, and family environments on the individual, thus always partially reasoned in terms of hereditary race linked to a fixed biological substrate. This conception of race enlightens us on how psychoanalysis was shaped in the United States, and the enduring importance attached to the biological nature of the individual. In the same article, Lind argued that black individuals often forgot dates and places, since their alleged mental deviance went hand in hand with their inability to behave responsibly in society. Making a general comment about his black patients' behavior, Lind argued that "it will often be found that a Negro is very poorly informed about the day of the month and the year," as "sometimes especially toward the end or the beginning of a month, he will give the following or the previous month instead of the correct one."

"The season, too is a rather indefinite division of time in his mind; he is very apt to base his answer on the state of the weather prevailing e.g., if it is a bright, balmy day in January or February, he will say it is spring; if the snow is falling in November, he will call it winter." Lind stated that the so-called child-like attitude of black patients affected their capacity to orientate themselves temporally. "Orientation for place and people is not apt to be at variance, but a Negro often spends from several days to several weeks in a hospital without bothering to ascertain its nomenclature accurately." Lind further recalled that when asked a question such as "Who is president of the United States?," his black patients "often bring forth the name of the last president instead of the present one, especially if the last president has a picturesque personality."

Here, Lind described the phenomenon of social disorientation experienced by patients interned often for long months, years even, isolated from society, yet he read into the phenomenon the signs of a biological and cultural difference between Whites and Blacks, thus pathologizing the poverty and marginality of these patients. Adopting the argument that race history weighed heavily on individual behavior, Lind believed that pathological behavior was due to "the frequent dissolution of families in slavery times, the tendency to license of all kinds immediately succeeding abolition," therefore issuing a moral judgment backed by medical expertise.

Quoting the founder of the journal, William Alanson White, about what constitutes a delusion in psychoanalysis, Lind warned his colleagues about possible misdiagnoses when confronted with black patients who were the victims of sensory hallucinations, thus insisting that different diagnoses be adopted according to the types of populations treated. "It is not surprising that the Negro, stocked as he is with the rich supply of traditions pertaining to haunts, night doctors, hags, and hoodoo men, which every old Negro uncle has at his command, should mistake things in dark and mysterious places for beings from another world, or that he should attribute persistent bad luck or ill health to evil influences of diabolical origin." Lind asked his fellow colleagues, when interacting with their black patients, to consider what he saw as a specific cultural heritage. "The most common error of all, perhaps, in dealing with the Negro, is to accept at its face value the statement that he has seen and talked with the Lord." Lind thus noted that black patients were particularly prone to religious fervor and advised his colleagues to "bear in mind, then, his credulity, his primitive reasoning powers, his superstitions, and his untrained observations."

Later in the text, Lind criticized the poor treatment of black individuals by the police, which led to major misunderstandings. "It sometimes happens here in Washington, DC, that Negroes arrive from country districts and almost immediately fall into the meshes of the police net through some absurd inquiry, or the statement that they have come to see the President to get some job," explained Lind, who described black men and black women as particularly credulous. "It develops then that the whole episode was the result of a practical joke by some town wag who told the Negro that all he had to do was to apply to the President in person and he would be accommodated." The psychiatrist further described how he saw the black population as infantile and naive regarding the jokes that targeted them. "Negroes have frequently been sent to the Government Hospital for the Insane, with some such statement as this: 'He thinks people are against him. Thinks people are putting a spell on him and trying to hoodoo him. Says some man burned some powder and this causes pain in his limbs.'"

Lind claimed scientific and moral authority over hospitalized black patients in his institution and concluded his article by giving specific advice to his colleagues: "Remember that his vocabulary is limited, that he does not speak your language. After you have decided that he actually does mean the statement as it is given, consider whether or not it is in accord with his psychology, his superstition, his prejudices, and his theology, in short, if it is what you would expect of a person whose great grandfather was perhaps a cannibal; and finally remember that, if after you have made a careful mental examination of a negro, and there is a doubt in your mind as to whether he is crazy or not, he probably is not."[53]

Authors in the *Psychoanalytic Review* not only commented upon what they saw as the black man's or woman's naïveté; they also coined new terms regarding a specific set of pathologies that designated the black patients' act of wanting to pass as white as a form of mental illness. In an article on the subject published in October 1914, Lind explained that Blacks were particularly prone to dementia, a condition caused by the stigma of not being white. The "color complex," as he called it, was defined as being based on the social subordination of the black man in the United States. Further on, Lind explained this "complex" by resorting to Freudian theories, especially wish fulfillment.

Freud had published his concept of wish fulfillment in 1899, in his book *Die Traumdeutung* (*The Interpretation of Dreams*), defining it as a response to the repression of desires. In his article, Lind applied this concept to Blacks who wished to pass as white in a society where there was a high improbability of crossing racial lines. Lind explained that Blacks were particularly prone to dementia caused by the stigma of not being white: "I have observed in the dreams of Negroes that frequently there will be presented some such dream picture as this, 'I saw my girl and she was white and talking to a lot of white people.'" Lind further commented that very often, "the dreamer finds himself in the company of white women or men who treat him as an equal," despite the dreamer being a black man. Lind reported that "usually in these instances, the dreamer adds the significant statement, 'I could not see what color I was myself.'"

To Lind, this was proof that psychiatrists had to accept "these dream pictures as wish-fulfillments, according to the Freudian doctrine," and he opined that they represented "further proofs of the repressed wishes present in the negro, i.e., to be white."[54] Later on in the same article, Lind quoted Austrian psychotherapist Alfred Adler, one of the most renowned figures in psychology and psychoanalysis in Europe at the time. Lind adopted Adler's theory of the inferiority complex and applied it to his black patients.

According to Adler, the inferiority complex stems from an adult's experience of being unable to reach a subconscious, reassuring, fictional final goal of subjective security. To Lind, black patients suffered from psychoses when they were in deep interaction with Whites, as feelings of inferiority grew within them. Lind thus applied Adler's theory, published in *Über den nervösen Charakter* (1912), to the context of racial segregation in the U.S. South.[55] Lind described cases in his hospital to show the plurality of diagnoses associated with the inferiority complex and the color complex, with the act of passing as an aggravating symptom.

In the first case, for example, Lind described a patient, A. W., who claimed to be a white man and suffered from dementia praecox. The patient was seen as being "unable to explain why he is not the same color as other white men but shows the palms of his hands which are very light colored and says that shows what his real color ought to be." To Lind, this patient suffered from the color complex, which he saw as the inability to cope with his own racial identity. "Asked if his parents were white, he says he never had a father or mother, but came into the world by himself." The patient's desire to pass as white was therefore medicalized by Lind.

In the second case, Lind also described a black patient, G. A., who wanted to pass as white and who suffered from this color complex because he "says he is white and that all his relatives were white." Lind reported that the patient "accounts for his present color by saying that dye in the water in which he washed changed his color" and that he "has often dreamed about doing business with white merchants who seemed to treat him as if he were a white man and their equal."

In the third case, Lind explored the life of a "paranoid dementia praecox" patient who held the belief that his ancestors were white and that therefore he could pass as white because "through his mother he descended from an Ethiopian prince who at one time conquered and ruled over Egypt." Lind explained that the patient believed that "the ancient Ethiopians . . . were not black but came from Eastern Asia and were light colored."[56]

In the same article, Lind mentioned his colleague Mary O'Malley, who was "in charge of the female department of the Government Hospital for the Insane, [who] assures me that the color complex is often found cropping out in the delusional field." O'Malley, a white woman, claimed to be a specialist, like Lind, in psychoses touching Blacks, and she had published the article "Psychoses in the Colored Race: A Study in Comparative Psychiatry" in the prestigious *American Journal of Insanity* in 1914.[57] Lind included O'Malley's patients' cases in his own article to further demonstrate the way in which the act of passing operated as a symptom of mental illness.

For example, he mentioned the case of A. L., a "paranoid praecox" patient who stated that "she is a white woman," and that "the present color of her skin has been caused by eating dark-colored food." Lind's use of this case demonstrates his willingness to confront and control the patient's desire to break free of racial constraints and classifications. Lind also cited another case, which for him was emblematic of the racial complex under discussion. Patient M. C. was "a colored male, aged 33, who [was] serving a life sentence for murder in the second degree." Lind explained that this patient's school life "lasted from his fifth to his sixteenth year," that "he has been a laborer," "has never married," and that "nothing abnormal sexually could be learned."

Lind reported that M. C. had been arrested and detained following a crime committed against another black man: "In 1907, at a negro picnic, he became involved in a quarrel with another negro over a woman and a bystander essayed the role of peacemaker." Lind reported that "the patient had an open knife in his hand with which he was cutting meat and, in the scuffle, stabbed the peacemaker, who afterwards died." M. C. was tried, convicted and sentenced to life imprisonment and arrived at the Leavenworth penitentiary in 1907. Soon after, in October 1912, M. C. was transferred to St. Elizabeths Hospital "on account of erratic behavior," where he was treated by Lind. The psychiatrist recalled that "M. C. called the attention of the prison physician to a tattoo mark on his hand and stated that he believed that he was not a negro but painted black," and that the patient claimed he had "a secret paint which he could use that would turn him white."

Interestingly enough for the understanding of the file, the patient, who apparently rejected his black status, was from the city of Washington, Louisiana, located in a rural parish where Blacks and Whites lived mixed. Lind indicated in his report that "if his townspeople in Washington, Louisiana, can be notified, the error would be rectified." The patient was undoubtedly also referring here to the very particular political situation in Louisiana, which unlike the other states of the Union during the nineteenth and early twentieth centuries, admitted very specific political and racial classifications. The black Creoles, for example, claimed mixed racial origins and thus represented a challenge to the one-drop rule, which usually classified populations in the United States in a binary way, physically separating Blacks from Whites in the South.

Placing the story of patient M. C. in this context, then, gives a new sense of causality to these episodes of delirium, which is hardly analyzed at all by Lind. if the patient in Louisiana had been used to passing for white or circulating in Louisiana society as a Creole—that is, if he was accustomed to adopting a different racial identity than black—and upon his arrival in Washington, DC, the patient was now, for the first time in his life, experiencing what it was like to be treated as a black man, it is quite possible that his behavioral disorders were also a mirror reflecting the change in treatment that he had to face. Although all the patients treated at the hospital suffered from particularly severe mental and behavioral disorders, psychiatrists paid particular attention to their patients' claims when they touched on questions of racial identity and the possibility of claiming or carrying out racial passing. The discourse of the patients was then analyzed by the doctors as unintelligible and ultimately irrelevant; they kept it at a distance because it revealed potential political stakes, as some of the patients attempted to break free of the racial classification that had been imposed on them.

In all of these cases, the act of passing—the willingness to pass as white and therefore to resist racial categorization—was pathologized by Lind, who saw whiteness as a superior form of identity that black patients wished for in order to be complete. Furthermore, Lind's racialist project highlighted the use of European psychoanalytic theories in the context of the segregated U.S. South. The local application of the color complex theory to the patients' cases in St. Elizabeths Hospital shows that Lind went beyond the theoretical framework proposed by Adler, since Lind mentioned "race" as the core element of his analysis.

As we have seen, after the period 1870 to 1880, southern psychiatric hospitals such as St. Elizabeths gradually began to consider the scientific and technological innovations that appeared on the international scene.[58] Consequently, southern hospitals underwent deep upheavals in the medicalization of black patients following the evolution of the rationalized international classifications. Nineteenth-century medical men were "moral entrepreneurs," as historian Andrew Scull defines them, because they shaped medical theories that took on broader symbolic significance in the society in which they were applied.[59]

The writings and pre-psychoanalytical frameworks of the physicians from Virginia, Louisiana, and North Carolina, such as Linville and Roberts, resonated strongly with the prose and theories developed at St. Elizabeths in Washington, DC, thus proving that a real continuum existed throughout the southern states, in terms of producing and applying in their public institutions (state or federal) epidemiological classifications based on race. Furthermore, as this chapter highlights, while black patients were understood as epidemiologically different from white patients in terms of treatment and research, these same black patients were no longer thought to be radically different when the opportunity arose for doctors to conduct medical experiments on black bodies for the purpose of advancing a so-called universalist science in fields such as child psychology.

The *Psychoanalytic Review* was an editorial platform that allowed the southern white physicians at St. Elizabeths to disseminate a model of psychiatry and psychoanalysis inherently built as a form of "political science" in the age of psychoanalysis. Furthermore, white psychoanalysts such as Evarts, Lind, and O'Malley were convinced that mental disorders affected Blacks and Whites differently, not only because of hereditary and biological causes rooted in bodies but also because of the different social environments in which the individuals had evolved in the South—including enslavement for Blacks and freedom for Whites. Psychiatrists paid particular attention to the issues of racial identity, sexuality, and their patients' ability to perform racial passing, thus giving us the best example of the tightly knit connections between state power and medical surveillance, or biopower.

Epidemiological differences were discussed only in relation to specific topics that all related, in one way or another, to the social, political, and moral order of the segregated South. A special emphasis was put on theories about primitivism (as when discussing suicide), sexual deviance, interracial relationships, the pathologization of mulattoes, and the act of passing as white, which was seen as a form of mental illness. Psychiatrists were seeking ways to control their patients' resistance to the racist social codes in place in the Jim Crow era. Therefore, paradoxically enough, the patients' words were thought by the doctors to be unintelligible and irrelevant, a mere side effect of their madness. Heard, but swiftly dismissed, the patients' claims were felt to be a site of resistance that held political stakes and that psychiatrists wanted to police and if possible, neutralize.

Psychiatry and psychoanalysis thus became inherently politicized sciences rooted in the age of Jim Crow, serving the interests of the white hegemony but also relying on a transnational global network of European and American psychoanalysts to orchestrate a transfer of knowledge and information about medical strategies to further discipline bodies, minds, and souls. These theories were then readapted to the local context, to the institutions in place, and gave rise to a new southern apparatus of science in the 1910s and onward, the aim of which was to discipline racialized bodies in their own local institutions.

EPILOGUE

An Everlasting Story: Race and Psychiatry in the United States Today

> History is not the past. It is the present.
> We carry our history with us. We are our history.
> —JAMES BALDWIN, in Raoul Peck,
> *I Am Not Your Negro*

In 1978, Todd Savitt, then assistant professor at the University of Florida College of Medicine, published his first book, *Medicine and Slavery: The Diseases and Health Care of Blacks in Antebellum Virginia*. When it came out, the book was something of a novelty in the field. In 2018, the book celebrated its thirtieth anniversary, and historians of slavery and of medicine now routinely praise its pioneering nature and its impact in this field of research over the years.[1] Savitt largely contributed to initiating research into the history of medical practices under slavery in relation to the construction and the perpetuation of a race-making system of oppression initiated by white power in the U.S. South.

As is true of other books dealing with the history of racial classifications in the medical field in the United States, this book owes a deep debt to *Medicine and Slavery*. It is fully in line with the historical approach built by Savitt, while renewing its challenges, and it proposes new perspectives to ensure the sustainability of a research field that is constantly growing.

First, this book sets out to reconcile the history of psychiatric institutions and the intellectual history of racial theories in psychiatry. As with Savitt's works, *Mad with Freedom* proposes a new reading of the history of medical theories and practices on plantations in the South, in relation to the concept of race, at the time of the beginning of the psychiatric profession in the United States in the 1840s. Many articles and historical works have focused on the development of various fields in racial medicine, including gynecological sciences, the resistance of enslaved people to white medical authority through the use of plant medicine, the links between polygenism and the Christian religion, medical experiments on the bodies of enslaved people, and general medicine. This book, however, has focused on the development of theories of madness in the South and its links with the history of slavery.

The progressive incursion of the race variable in treating madness gave rise to specific medical theories about pathologies affecting supposedly white and black brains in different ways. These theories, which emerged mainly in medical schools in the South, such as at the Medical Department of the University of Louisiana (formerly the Medical College of Louisiana), had the wind in their sails in the 1860s, when anti-abolitionists took up the medical argument that freedmen would be affected by madness when faced with the complexities of freedom. The white southern power relied on local medical personalities and their networks (including doctors in the rural countryside of the South, teachers of medicine in the new training courses for doctors, and publications promoting the writings of southern doctors) to expand and spread the idea of a mental and moral inferiority of Blacks compared to Whites, which, according to white physicians, made them naturally unfit for freedom.

Moreover, as we saw in chapters 3 and 4, white medical professionals sought to medicalize black bodies as idle and lazy compared to white workers, even while the medical profession considered them to be particularly suitable for the physical work of plantations. This further demonstrates that the medicalization of stolen black labor for the profits of landowners, both in the antebellum and postbellum eras, was part of an effort to legitimize black bodily inferiority and the southern social order. This book has proposed to give greater space to reflections on the history of medicine and race, with a view to emphasizing the need to take into account both social history and sociology to apprehend questions relating to civil rights and the social control of populations in the United States.

The second aim of this book has been to deal with a period much less studied than the slavery period in the historiography of medicine, namely, the post–Civil War era and Reconstruction, by examining the massive institutionalization of Blacks in segregated asylums or psychiatric hospitals built specifically for this population in the New South from the 1870s onward. This movement to institutionalize black patients resulted in an increasing contact between white doctors and black patients. The experiences of the very first black patients admitted to psychiatric institutions in the South after the 1870s is traced using mainly three case studies from hospitals in Virginia, North Carolina, and Louisiana.

The book also explored the emergence of a classification system of pathologies developed in the South to differentiate black and white patients in these same institutions, and the routines organized by white physicians to constrain black bodies in separate spaces. It turns out that the classification system of black patients in the Jim Crow era was modeled on and came to perpetuate, in the South, previous theories that had emerged since the 1840s about the spread of madness among free Blacks, thus providing tangible proof of the continued politicization of psychiatry at the time of white political and social hegemony. The book also revealed the continuity and divergences between pre-Freudian theories on blackness and madness and the advent of psychoanalysis in the United States, which gave rise to reformulated analyses of primitivism, barbarism, and sexual deviance.

Overall, this book has united an institutional history of asylums and hospitals in several states in the South with a history of treatments, practices, and theories developed by white physicians, in order to analyze the broader medical racialized apparatus from 1840 to 1930. In a way, therefore, *Mad with Freedom* proposes to reconcile two visions of history: the first apprehending historical facts as if they concerned another country, theorizing history as a past moment dissociated from the contemporary and irreconcilable with the present; and the second apprehending history as a living element in each of us.

In many ways, each chapter and the themes with which they deal are connected to a broader contemporary social agenda. Despite the fact that disciplines and academic fields very often are described as nonporous, based on different methodologies (archival research, qualitative fieldwork, and so on) and different approaches, discussing themes such as racial discrimination and medical treatments is useful in shaping a continuum between past and present oppressions. Historians of science and scholars of black history should not be surprised to encounter useful information and arguments ostensibly outside their period in books and articles that deal with contemporary health trends and racial disparities, in fields such as the anthropology of medicine or the sociology of science.

For example, recently published articles in the social sciences reveal racial bias in diagnoses, and by extension in drug prescriptions, when psychiatrists— who in the United States are predominantly white—treat racialized patients today.[2] These works, whether based on qualitative or quantitative studies, further demonstrate the persistence of patterns of racial differentiation, discrimination, and systemic racism in health care today. Similarly, social historian Mical Raz and medical anthropologist Philippe Bourgois have demonstrated how the successive public policies of the neoliberal era, since the end of the 1970s, have impacted relentlessly and in a negative way the psychiatric care offered to racialized populations who are vulnerable in terms of socioeconomics. Mical Raz's work has revealed the history of the gradual medicalization of black poverty since the 1960s, while anthropologists Helena Hansen and Philippe Bourgois along with epidemiologist Ernest Drucker have addressed the consequences of the closure of public psychiatric care centers in California for racialized populations, which have suffered the most from budget cuts and a drastic lack of care.[3]

Throughout the twentieth century, medical institutions such as psychiatric hospitals and prisons have indeed become communicating vessels, in an era in which the federal, state, and local governments have withdrawn public funding from health care facilities and public education, due to the advent of neoliberal policies that have repeatedly and consistently chipped away at the welfare state.[4] This situation has gained much media attention in recent years, since the Black Lives Matter movement and other progressive activist organizations have alerted us to the deadly consequences of a public policy apparatus that substitutes police brutality and mass incarceration for black mental health care.

These topics of analysis (social control, racialization processes, the deterioration of public funding for welfare institutions for black patients, an overwhelming lack of diversity in medical personnel, and differential treatments in health care institutions) are therefore contiguous to those dealt with in *Mad with Freedom*, despite the focus on different centuries and local configurations. This permanence, this persistence, can only encourage historians and scholars in the social sciences to shape a new public history and sociology of race and medicine, in order to form a critical viewpoint. There is no doubt that the story that is told in this book will continue to resonate with present situations and will stimulate further debate regarding health care disparities and race in the twenty-first century.

Notes

Introduction

1. Throughout this book, I have capitalized the racial categories White and Black when they are nouns. White physicians employed other terms to describe black patients. These terms denote the derogatory and offensive attitudes that white officials held toward their patients. I have purposefully chosen to not employ such terms unless as an object of analysis when they are displayed in quotes. In an effort not to essentialize through the use of biased language, I employ the terms *enslaved people/the enslaved, enslaver,* and *fugitives from slavery* instead of *slaves, slaveholders,* and *runaway slaves.* I have purposefully chosen not to use the term *care* when referring to the treatment of black individuals by white personnel or institutions.

2. See Joseph Crespino, *In Search of Another Country: Mississippi and the Conservative Counterrevolution* (Princeton, NJ: Princeton University Press, 2007), 144; and M. J. O'Brien, *We Shall Not Be Moved: The Jackson Woolworth's Sit-In and the Movement It Inspired* (Jackson: University Press of Mississippi, 2013), 180.

3. James Baldwin, *I Am Not Your Negro: A Major Motion Picture Directed by Raoul Peck* (New York: Vintage Books, 2017), 98.

4. Jonathan Metzl, *The Protest Psychosis: How Schizophrenia Became a Black Disease* (Boston: Beacon Press, 2011). For psychiatry, blackness, and social control in the 1960s, see Élodie Edwards-Grossi, *Bad Brains: La psychiatrie et la lutte des Noirs américains pour la justice raciale, XXe–XXIe siècles* (Rennes: Presses universitaires de Rennes, 2021).

5. See also Felicia Pride, "Schizophrenia as Political Weapon," *The Root,* January 25, 2010.

6. Metzl, *Protest Psychosis.*

7. For a denunciation of these stereotypes, see Audre Lorde, "The Uses of Anger: Women Responding to Racism" (June 1981), *Black Past,* August 12, 2012. See also Brittney Cooper, *Eloquent Rage: A Black Feminist Discovers Her Superpower* (New York: St. Martin's Press, 2018).

8. For psychiatry as a means of social control, see Michel Foucault, *Histoire de la Folie à l'Age Classique* (Paris: Gallimard, 1972); Robert Castel, *L'Ordre psychiatrique* (Paris: Éditions de Minuit, 1976); Thomas Szasz, *The Myth of Mental Illness* (New York: Hoeber-Harper, 1961); Mark Micale and Roy Porter, *Discovering the History of Psychiatry* (Oxford: Oxford University Press, 1994); David Rothman, *The Discovery of the Asylum: Social Order and Disorder in the New Republic* (Boston: Little, Brown, 1971); Erving Goffman, *Asylums: Essays on the Social Situation of Mental Patients and Other Inmates* (Chicago: Aldine Transaction, 1968); and Gerald Grob, *Mad Among Us* (New York: Simon and Schuster, 1994).

9. See William Stanton, *The Leopard's Spots: Scientific Attitudes Toward Race in America, 1815–59* (Chicago: University of Chicago Press, 1960); and Alexander Thomas and Samuel Sillen, *Racism and Psychiatry* (New York: Brunner/Mazel, 1972). See also Sander L. Gilman, *Difference and Pathology: Stereotypes of Sexuality, Race, and Madness* (Ithaca, NY: Cornell University Press, 1985).

10. See Metzl, *Protest Psychosis*.

11. See Dennis Doyle, *Psychiatry and Racial Liberalism in Harlem, 1936–1968* (Rochester, NY: University of Rochester Press, 2016); Gabriel N. Mendes, *Under the Strain of Color: Harlem's Lafargue Clinic and the Promise of an Antiracist Psychiatry* (Ithaca, NY: Cornell University Press, 2015); Mical Raz, *What's Wrong with the Poor? Psychiatry, Race, and the War on Poverty* (Chapel Hill: University of North Carolina Press, 2013). For race, medicine, and segregation in the twentieth century, see Karen Kruse Thomas, *Deluxe Jim Crow: Civil Rights and American Health Policy, 1935–1954* (Athens: University of Georgia Press, 2011).

12. See Manuella Meyer, *Reasoning Against Madness: Psychiatry and the State in Rio de Janeiro, 1830–1944* (Rochester, NY: University of Rochester Press, 2017); Jim Downs, *Maladies of Empire: How Colonialism, Slavery, and War Transformed Medicine* (Cambridge, MA: Harvard University Press, 2021); Delphine Peiretti-Courtis, *Corps noirs et médecins blancs: La fabrique du préjugé racial, XIXe–XXe siècles* (Paris: La Découverte, 2021); Sean Morey Smith and Christopher D. E. Willoughby, eds., *Medicine and Healing in the Age of Slavery* (Baton Rouge: Louisiana State University Press, 2021). For recent works about slavery from a past and present perspective, see Ana Lucia Araujo, *Museums and Atlantic Slavery* (New York: Routledge, 2020); and Ana Lucia Araujo, *Slavery in the Age of Memory: Engaging the Past* (New York: Bloomsbury, 2020).

13. Sharla M. Fett, *Working Cures: Healing, Health, and Power on Southern Slave Plantations* (Chapel Hill: University of North Carolina Press, 2002); Londa Schiebinger, *Secret Cures of Slaves: People, Plants, and Medicine in the Eighteenth-Century Atlantic World* (Palo Alto, CA: Stanford University Press, 2017).

14. Stephen C. Kenny, "'A Dictate of Both Interest and Mercy'? Slave Hospitals in the Antebellum South," *Journal of the History of Medicine and Allied Sciences* 65, no. 1 (January 2010): 2–47; Kenny, "The Development of Medical Museums in the Antebellum American South: Slave Bodies in Networks of Anatomical Exchange," *Bulletin of the History of Medicine* 87, no. 1 (Spring 2013): 32–62; Kenny, "Power, Opportunism, Racism: Human Experiments Under American Slavery," *Endeavour* 39, no. 1 (2015): 10–20; Deirdre Cooper Owens, *Medical Bondage: Race, Gender, and the Origins of American Gynecology* (Athens: University of Georgia Press, 2016); Rana Hogarth, *Medicalizing Blackness: Making Racial Difference in the Atlantic World, 1780–1840* (Chapel Hill: University of North Carolina Press, 2017); Vincent Woodard, *The Delectable Negro: Human Consumption and Homoeroticism Within U.S. Slave Culture* (New York: New York University Press, 2014); Daina Ramey Berry, *The Price for Their Pound of Flesh: The Value of the Enslaved, from Womb to the Grave, in the Building of a Nation* (Boston: Beacon Press, 2017).

15. On Samuel Cartwright, see Christopher Willoughby, "Running Away from Drapetomania: Samuel Cartwright, Medicine, and Race in the Antebellum South," *Journal of Southern History* 84, no. 3 (August 2018): 579–614. On James Babcock, see Charles S. Bryan, *Asylum Doctor: James Woods Babcock and the Red Plague of Pellagra* (Columbia: University of South Carolina Press, 2014).

16. Jim Downs, *Sick from Freedom: African-American Illness and Suffering During the Civil War and Reconstruction* (Oxford: Oxford University Press, 2012): 4–7. For more on slavery, health, and the Civil War, see Gretchen Long, *Doctoring Freedom: The Politics of African American Medical Care in Slavery and Emancipation* (Chapel Hill: University of North Carolina Press, 2012); and Margaret Humphreys, *Intensely Human: The Health of the Black Soldier in the American Civil War* (Baltimore: Johns Hopkins University Press, 2008).

17. Pippa Holloway, *Sexuality, Politics, and Social Control in Virginia, 1920–1945* (Chapel Hill: University of North Carolina Press, 2006).

18. See Peter McCandless, *Slavery, Disease, and Suffering in the Southern Low Country* (Cambridge: Cambridge University Press, 2011).

19. Mab Segrest, *Administrations of Lunacy: Racism and the Haunting of American Psychiatry at the Milledgeville Asylum* (New York: The New Press, 2020); Wendy Gonaver, *The Peculiar Institution and the Making of Modern Psychiatry, 1840–1880* (Chapel Hill: University of North Carolina Press, 2019); Martin Summers, *Madness in the City of Magnificent Intentions: A History of Race and Mental Illness in the Nation's Capital* (New York: Oxford University Press, 2019). See also Summers, "Diagnosing the Ailments of Black Citizenship: The African American Medical Profession and the Politics of Mental Illness, 1895–1940," in *Precarious Prescriptions: Contested Histories of Race and Health in North America,* ed. Laurie Green, John McKiernan-Gonzalez, and Martin Summers, 91–114 (Minneapolis: University of Minnesota Press, 2014).

20. Segrest, *Administrations of Lunacy,* introduction.

21. On sexual deviance, see Holloway, *Sexuality, Politics, and Social Control.*

22. These works include Keith Wailoo, *Dying in the City of the Blues: Sickle Cell Anemia and the Politics of Race and Health* (Chapel Hill: University of North Carolina Press, 2014); John Hoberman, *Black and Blue: The Origins and Consequences of Medical Racism* (Berkeley: University of California Press, 2012); Harriet A. Washington, *Medical Apartheid: The Dark History of Medical Experimentation on Black Americans from Colonial Times to the Present* (New York: Knopf Doubleday, 2008); and Gregory Michael Dorr, *Segregation's Science: Eugenics and Society in Virginia* (Charlottesville: University of Virginia Press, 2008).

23. See, for example, Doyle, *Psychiatry and Racial Liberalism.*

24. It would be impossible to identify all the public and private asylums existing in the United States over the period. However, by 1870, all the southern states had at least one asylum and had made arrangements to treat both white and black patients. Some institutions were segregated; others welcomed only Whites or only Blacks. Chapter 3 will cover this issue.

25. See Segrest, *Administrations of Lunacy.*

26. Michael Burawoy, "For Public Sociology," *American Sociological Review* 70, no. 1 (February 2005): 4–28.

1. The "Sane Slaves": Theories about Madness and Blackness, 1800–1860

1. Dorothea Dix, *Memorial Soliciting Enlarged and Improved Accommodations for the Establishment of a New Hospital for the Insane of the State of Tennessee* (Nashville: General Assembly Press, 1847), 1.

2. See Dorothea Dix, "Memorial to the Massachusetts Legislature (1843)," https://usa
.usembassy.de/etexts/democrac/15.htm; Manon Parry, "Dorothea Dix," *American Journal of
Public Health* 96 (April 2006): 624–625; Francis Tiffany, *Life of Dorothea Lynde Dix* (Boston:
Houghton, Mifflin, 1890), 134–149; and Tamonud Modak, Siddharth Sarkar, and Rajesh Sagar,
"Dorothea Dix: A Proponent of Humane Treatment of Mentally Ill," *Journal of Mental Health
and Human Behaviour* 21 (January 2016): 69–71.

3. On the living conditions of patients in European asylums in the nineteenth century, see
Lydie Couturier, "L'enfermement des aliénés: l'asile de Stephansfeld (Bas-Rhin, 1835–1860) et la
loi de 1838," *Revue d'Histoire de la Protection Sociale* 7, no. 1 (January 2014): 58–79.

4. Dix, *Memorial Soliciting Enlarged and Improved Accommodations,* 5.

5. Numerous enslaved people lived on plantations in the state of Tennessee. See, for example,
Larry McKee, "The Archaeological Study of Slavery and Plantation Life in Tennessee," *Tennes-
see Historical Quarterly* 59, no. 3 (Fall 2000): 188–203. On Native Americans, see Ronald Satz,
Tennessee's Indian Peoples: From White Contact to Removal, 1540–1840 (Knoxville: University of
Tennessee Press, 1979).

6. On the Second Middle Passage, see Thavolia Glymph, "The Second Middle Passage: The
Transition from Slavery to Freedom at Davis Bend, Mississippi" (PhD diss., Purdue University,
1994).

7. See Leonard A. Carlson and Mark A. Roberts, "Indian Lands, 'Squatterism,' and Slavery:
Economic Interests and the Passage of the Indian Removal Act of 1830," *Explorations in Economic
History* 43, no. 3 (2006): 486–504.

8. The racial and geographic classifications of intelligence and morality adopted by Carl von
Linné, a Swedish naturalist, are some of the first examples of classifications of this type in the
eighteenth century. See Nicholas Hudson, "From 'Nation' to 'Race': The Origin of Racial Classification in Eighteenth-Century Thought," *Eighteenth-Century Studies* 29, no. 3 (Spring 1996):
247–264; and Londa Schiebinger, "The Anatomy of Difference: Race and Sex in Eighteenth-
Century Science," *Eighteenth-Century Studies* 23, no. 4 (Summer 1990): 387–405.

9. Chapter 2 of historian Ellen Dwyer's *Sex Roles and Psychopathology* says that the first
writings of Benjamin Rush on madness date back to 1812. However, while consulting the B. Rush
papers at the Library of Congress in Washington, DC, I found a scrapbook from 1804 that belonged to Rush, to which he consigned various conference notes from Philadelphia about diseases of the mind and insanity. Dwyer, "A Historical Perspective," in *Sex Roles and Psychopathology,* ed. Cathy Widom (Berlin: Springer, 2013), 21; Benjamin Rush, "Syllabus of a Course of
Lectures upon Physiology, Pathology, Therapeutics and Practice of Medicine, vol. 1," 1804, in
Benjamin Rush papers, 1776–1812, Manuscript Division, MSS38547, Library of Congress, Washington, DC.

10. Benjamin Rush, *Medical Inquiries and Observations upon the Diseases of the Mind* (Philadelphia: Kimber & Richardson, 1812), 41. Also mentioned in Pedro Ruiz and Annelle Primm,
eds., *Disparities in Psychiatric Care: Clinical and Cross-Cultural Perspectives,* (Baltimore: Lippincott Williams & Wilkins, 2010), 14.

11. See Edward Allen Driggers, "The Chemistry of Blackness: Benjamin Rush, Thomas Jefferson, Everard Home, and the Project of Defining Blackness Through Chemical Explanations,"
Critical Philosophy of Race 7, no. 2 (July 2019): 372–391.

12. On leprosy, see Winthrop D. Jordan, *White over Black: American Attitudes Toward the Negro, 1550–1812* (Chapel Hill: University of North Carolina Press, 2013), 523–525. On black leprosy, see Andy Doolen, *Fugitive Empire: Locating Early American Imperialism* (Minneapolis: University of Minnesota Press, 2005), 71.

13. See Samuel Stanhope Smith, *Essay on the Causes of Variety of Complexion and Figure in the Human Species* (New Brunswick: L. Simpson & Co., 1810). Smith was a fierce advocate of the environmental model. According to him, racial characteristics diverge as they have evolved with the environment. For monogenism, see Charles Caldwell, *Thoughts on the Original Unity of the Human Race* (Cincinnati: J. A. & U. P. James, 1852); and George M. Fredrickson, *The Black Image in the White Mind: The Debate on Afro-American Character and Destiny, 1817–1914* (New York: Harper & Row, 1971).

14. For an obituary of Samuel G. Morton with a summary of his works, see Charles D. Meigs, "Article XII: Extract from a Memoir of Samuel George Morton, M.D., Late President of the Academy of Natural Sciences of Philadelphia," *American Journal of Science* 13, no. 38 (May 1852): 153–178.

15. Samuel George Morton, *Crania Americana: or, a Comparative View of the Skulls of Various Aboriginal Nations of North and South America* (Philadelphia: J. Dobson, 1839); Morton, *Crania Ægyptiaca: Observations on Egyptian Ethnography, Derived from Anatomy, History and the Monuments* (Philadelphia: John Pennington, 1844); Morton, *An Inquiry into the Distinctive Characteristics of the Aboriginal Race of America* (Philadelphia: John Pennington, 1844).

16. Thomas Jefferson, *Notes on the State of Virginia* (London: John Stockdale, 1787).

17. See Frank Luther Mott, *A History of American Magazines, 1850–1865* (Cambridge, MA: Harvard University Press, 1938), 84; and Joseph Garland, "The Boston Medical and Surgical Journal, 1828–1928," *New England Journal of Medicine* 198, no. 1 (January 1928): 1–13. Using the HathiTrust Digital Library, I made a survey of all articles published between 1810 and 1840 with the words *colored, black,* or *slave,* correlated with the term *insanity.*

18. See *New England Journal of Medicine* 1 (February 19, 1828–February 10, 1829): 111; 6–7 (1832–1833): 112–115 and 397; 13 (1835–1836): 187; 15–16 (1836–1837): 27; 18 (1838): 235; and 20 (1839): 331. Most of these medical case reports are presented in the form of first-person accounts—the physician in charge usually gives details of a specific treatment and then the autopsy results (in cases where the treatment has failed)—while others are in the form of succinct institutional reports.

19. On the diseases, symptoms, and treatments prescribed to enslaved people on antebellum plantations, see Katherine Bankole-Medina, *Slavery and Medicine: Enslavement and Medical Practices in Antebellum Louisiana* (New York: Taylor and Francis, 1998), appendixes A, B, C and D.

20. See Cartwright's eulogy in Mary Louise Marshall, "Samuel A. Cartwright and States' Rights Medicine," *New Orleans Medical and Surgical Journal* 90 (August 1940): 74–78; and in Samuel Adolphus Cartwright 1793–1863 Family Papers [Cartwright Family Papers], Mss. 2471, 2499, box 1, folder 5, Louisiana and Lower Mississippi Valley Collections, LSU Libraries Special Collections, Hill Memorial Library, Louisiana State University, Baton Rouge.

21. For polygenism, see "Unity of the Human Race Disproved by the Hebrew Bible," *De Bow's Review* 4, no. 2 (August 1860): 129–136, in Cartwright Family Papers, box 1, folder 5 (printed pamphlets). Some historians mention that Cartwright studied at the University of Pennsylvania

under the aegis of Benjamin Rush, but there is no positive evidence to suggest that this is based on fact. See Bob Myers, "Drapetomania: Rebellion, Defiance and Free Black Insanity in the Antebellum United States" (PhD diss., University of California Los Angeles, 2014).

22. Christopher D. E. Willoughby, "Running Away from Drapetomania: Samuel A. Cartwright, Medicine, and Race in the Antebellum South," *Journal of Southern History* 84 (August 2018): 579–614; Steven M. Stowe, *Doctoring the South: Southern Physicians and Everyday Medicine in the Mid-Nineteenth Century* (Chapel Hill: University of North Carolina Press, 2004), 216; Stephen C. Kenny, "The Development of Medical Museums in the Antebellum American South: Slave Bodies in Networks of Anatomical Exchange," *Bulletin of the History of Medicine* 87 (Spring 2013): 32–62; Kenny, "Medical Racism's Poison Pen: The Toxic World of Dr. Henry Ramsay (1821–1856)," *Southern Quarterly* 53 (Spring–Summer 2016): 70–96; Eugene Genovese, *Roll, Jordan, Roll: The World the Slaves Made* (New York: Vintage, 1976); John S. Haller Jr., "The Negro and the Southern Physician: A Study of Medical and Racial Attitudes, 1800–1860," *Medical History* 16 (July 1972): 238–253.

23. See *Boston Medical and Surgical Journal* (August 22, 1849): 63–64; and "Letter from John Gorham to Samuel Cartwright," August 10, 1826, in Cartwright Family Papers, box 1, folder 1 (1826–1850). Cartwright received many medals and medical awards. The Medical and Chirurgical Faculty of Maryland gave him a $100 prize for his essay on cholera infantum. He received a medal from the Harvard Boylston Medical Committee and a prize from the Baltimore Medical Society. It is interesting to note that he was invited by the medical faculty of Paris, and that his treatise on yellow fever was translated and praised by the French government, which also gave an international scope to his career.

24. See "Letter from the Deinologian Society," in Cartwright Family Papers, box 1, file 1 (1826–1850). The Deinologian Society was very active, especially in Kentucky, in supporting the advent of southern universities whose religious and political teachings were favorable to anti-abolitionism. On this matter, see Alfred Brophy, *University, Court, and Slave: Pro-slavery Thought in Southern Colleges and Courts and the Coming of Civil War* (Oxford: Oxford University Press, 2016).

25. Marshall, "Samuel A. Cartwright," 78.

26. "Letter from Dr. Cartwright to Dr. Joseph S. Copes," February 22, 1848, box 7, file 14, Joseph S. Copes Papers 1831–1936, collection 733, Louisiana Research Collection, Tulane University, New Orleans.

27. Marshall, "Samuel A. Cartwright," 78.

28. Samuel A. Cartwright, "Report on the Diseases and Physical Peculiarities of the Negro Race," *New Orleans Medical and Surgical Journal* 7 (May 1851): 703.

29. S. L. Grier, "The Negro and His Diseases," *New Orleans Medical and Surgical Journal* 9 (January 1853): 752. See also Dea H. Boster, *African American Slavery and Disability: Bodies, Property, and Power in the Antebellum South, 1800–1860* (New York: Routledge, 2014); and Nancy Krieger, "Shades of Difference: Theoretical Underpinnings of the Medical Controversy on Black/White Differences in the United States 1830–1870," *International Journal of Health Services* 17, no. 2 (January 1987): 259–278.

30. Grier, "The Negro and His Diseases," 762.

31. For southern distinctiveness, see, for example, Frederick H. Siegel's classic book in his-

torical sociology. Siegel, *The Roots of Southern Distinctiveness: Tobacco and Society in Danville, Virginia, 1780–1865* (Chapel Hill: University of North Carolina Press, 1987).

32. See Scott R. Meinke, "Slavery, Partisanship, and Procedure in the U.S. House: The Gag Rule, 1836–1845," *Legislative Studies Quarterly* 32, no. 1 (2007): 33–58.

33. Sarah Bischoff Paulus, "America's Long Eulogy for Compromise: Henry Clay and American Politics, 1854–58," *Journal of the Civil War Era* 4, no. 1 (2014): 28–52.

34. Willoughby, "Running Away from Drapetomania," 592.

35. "Letter from Henry Clay to Cartwright," October 14, 1844, in Cartwright Family Papers, box 1, file 1a (1826–1849).

36. See "Letter from Jefferson Davis to Cartwright," September 23, 1851, and January 20, 1853, in Cartwright Family Papers, box 1, file 2 (1851–1853). See also "Personal Letter from Jefferson Davis to General Joseph Eggleston Johnston," June 9, 1861, box 11, file 53, Kuntz Collection, Collection 600, Louisiana Research Collection, Tulane University, New Orleans, in which Jefferson Davis introduces him to Cartwright.

37. "Letter from Jefferson Davis to Cartwright," June 10, 1849, box 1, file 1a (1826–1849), Cartwright Family Papers.

38. "Letter from Quitman to Cartwright," October 2, 1850, box 1, file 1b (1850) Cartwright Family Papers.

39. See "Letter from G. W. Marshall to Cartwright," August 30, 1853, box 1, file 2 (1851–1853), Cartwright Family Papers.

40. "Letter from Dr. Marshall to Cartwright," October 23, 1854, box 1, file 2 (1851–1853), Cartwright Family Papers.

41. Samuel Cartwright, "Ethnology of the Negro or Prognathous Race," New Orleans Academy of Sciences, November 30, 1857, published in the *New Orleans Medical and Surgical Journal* 15 (January 1858): 149–163.

42. Steve Deyle, *Carry Me Back: The Domestic Slave Trade in American Life* (New York: Oxford University Press, 2005), 289. See also Walter Johnson, *River of Dark Dreams: Slavery and Empire in the Cotton Kingdom* (Cambridge, MA: Belknap Press of Harvard University Press, 2013); Erskine Clarke, *Dwelling Place: A Plantation Epic* (New Haven, CT: Yale University Press, 2005); and Ira Berlin, *Generations of Captivity: A History of African-American Slaves* (Cambridge, MA: Belknap Press of Harvard University Press, 2003).

43. On the 1830 U.S. census, see *Abstract of the Returns of the Fifth Census* (Washington, DC: Duff Green, 1832). For the 1850 U.S. census, see J. D. B. De Bow, *Statistical View of the United States* (Washington, DC: Beverley Tucker, Senate Printer, 1854).

44. Carlson and Roberts, "Indian Lands."

45. Richard J. Blackett, "Dispossessing Massa: Fugitive Slaves and the Politics of Slavery After 1850," *American Nineteenth Century History* 10, no. 2 (2009): 119–136.

46. See John Wesley Monette, *An Essay on Causes of the Variety of Complexion and Form of the Human Species,* 1824, Mss. 593, Louisiana and Lower Mississippi Valley Collections, LSU Libraries Special Collections, Louisiana State University Libraries, Baton Rouge.

47. See Genovese, *Roll, Jordan, Roll,* 295. Genovese mentions Cartwright at the end of the chapter to show the contradictions between the two types of arguments raised by white enslavers who describe laziness—or on the contrary, the laborious nature—of enslaved people.

48. Frederick Law Olmsted, *A Journey in the Back Country* (New York: Mason Brothers, 1860), 228–229. W. E. B. Du Bois brings a culturalist explanation to clarify the ethical differences between white and black workers. According to him, the white people's ethos, which would explain their greater efficiency, had been influenced by Europeans and their capitalist system, while black individuals in the United States had inherited customs from forms of collectivist labor organization. Du Bois, *The Gift of Black Folk: The Negroes in the Making of America* (Oxford: Oxford University Press, 2009), 308.

49. Peter McCandless, *Moonlight, Magnolias, and Madness: Insanity in South Carolina from the Colonial Period to the Progressive Era* (Chapel Hill: University of North Carolina Press, 1996); Todd Savitt, *Medicine and Slavery: The Diseases and Health Care of Blacks in Antebellum Virginia* (Champaign: University of Illinois Press, 1978); Marli F. Weiner and Mazie Hough, *Sex, Sickness, and Slavery: Illness in the Antebellum South* (Champaign: University of Illinois Press, 2012).

50. See Bankole-Medina, *Slavery and Medicine*, 8; Rana Hogarth, *Medicalizing Blackness: Making Racial Difference in the Atlantic World, 1780–1840* (Chapel Hill: University of North Carolina Press, 2017); Deirdre Cooper Owens, *Medical Bondage: Race, Gender, and the Origins of American Gynecology* (Athens: University of Georgia Press, 2016); Vincent Woodard, *The Delectable Negro: Human Consumption and Homoeroticism Within U.S. Slave Culture* (New York: New York University Press, 2014); and Daina Ramey Berry, *The Price for Their Pound of Flesh: The Value of the Enslaved, from Womb to Grave, in the Building of a Nation* (Boston: Beacon Press, 2017).

51. Willoughby, "Running Away from Drapetomania," 606.

52. Cartwright, "Ethnology of the Negro or Prognathous Race."

53. See Junius P. Rodriguez, "Always 'En Garde': The Effects of Slave Insurrection upon the Louisiana Mentality, 1811–1815," *Louisiana History: The Journal of the Louisiana Historical Association* 33, no. 4 (Autumn 1992): 399–416.

54. See Harvey Wish, "The Slave Insurrection Panic of 1856," *Journal of Southern History* 5, no. 2 (May 1939): 217.

55. See McCandless, *Moonlight, Magnolias, and Madness*, 15.

56. A law of 1717 had created a fine of twenty pounds for anyone who refused to make arrangements for the care of enslaved people who were sick or disabled.

57. Orlando Patterson, *Slavery and Social Death: A Comparative Study* (Cambridge, MA: Harvard University Press, 1982), 38–45.

58. See Philip Morgan, *Slave Counterpoint: Black Culture in the Eighteenth-Century Chesapeake and Low Country* (Chapel Hill: University of North Carolina Press, 1998), 323–324; Gretchen Long, *Doctoring Freedom: The Politics of African American Medical Care in Slavery and Emancipation* (Chapel Hill: University of North Carolina Press, 2016); and Sharla Fett, *Working Cures: Healing, Health, and Power on Southern Slave Plantations* (Chapel Hill: University of North Carolina Press, 2002).

59. See Stephanie Jones-Rogers, "'She could . . . spare one ample breast for the profit of her owner': White Mothers and Enslaved Wet Nurses' Invisible Labor in American Slave Markets," *Slavery & Abolition* 38, no. 2 (2017): 1–19.

60. See Fett, *Working Cures*, 15–35.

61. "Cancellation of contract to sell slave an agreement between Joseph Brunei and Edouard

Rieffel, both of NO," November 18, 1847, Kuntz collection, III. National period, box 10, file 25, Louisiana Research Collection, Tulane University, New Orleans.

62. Stanford Emerson Chaillé, *A Memoir of the Insane Asylum of the State of Louisiana, at Jackson* (Baton Rouge, LA: J. M. Taylor, 1858), 9.

63. See Morgan, *Slave Counterpoint,* 323.

64. On the Eastern Lunatic Asylum, see "Appendix: Miscellaneous Items Relative to the Colored Insane (with notes)," box 29, file 4, undated; and "Committee Appointed on Asylums for Colored People—Report to the Association of Medical Superintendents of American Institutions for the Insane, undated (post-1844)," box 29, file 43, in Subseries D. Correspondence, Subject Files and Ledgers (Superintendent) 1791–1937, Eastern State Hospital Collection, Library of Virginia, Richmond. On the care of black patients by asylums more generally, see Gerald Grob, *Mental Institutions in America: Social Policy to 1875* (New York: Free Press, 1973), 243–255; Savitt, *Medicine and Slavery,* 258–279; Norman Dain, *Disordered Minds: The First Century of Eastern State Hospital in Williamsburg, Virginia, 1766–1866* (Charlottesville: University Press of Virginia, 1971), 19; and Dain, *Concepts of Insanity in the United States, 1789–1865* (New Brunswick, NJ: Rutgers University Press, 1964), 107–108. On John Galt at the Eastern Lunatic Asylum and Francis Stribling at the Western Lunatic Asylum, another facility in Virginia, see also Constance McGovern, *Masters of Madness: Social Origins of the American Psychiatric Profession* (Burlington: University of Vermont Press, 1985), 69.

65. "Notes on Admission of Colored Patients," undated letter, Eastern State Hospital Collection, Subseries D. Correspondence, Subject Files and Ledgers (Superintendent), 1791–1937, box 28, file 22, Virginia State Archives, Library of Virginia, Richmond. A third hospital for Whites, the Southwestern State Hospital, opened in Virginia in 1887, and in 1921 a special unit opened to treat mentally ill criminals and white patients.

66. "They are hereby empowered to receive into the said asylum insane slaves as patients on applications of their owners or of others having said slaves in charge." Wendy Gonaver, *The Peculiar Institution and the Making of Modern Psychiatry, 1840–1880* (Chapel Hill: University of North Carolina Press, 2019), 5.

67. "Remarks respecting a proposed law prohibiting the Western Asylum from making selection as to cases applying for admission to that institution," undated, box 32, file 19, Subseries D. Correspondence, Subject Files and Ledgers (Superintendent), 1791–1937, Eastern State Hospital Collection, Library of Virginia, Richmond.

68. "Admission of insane slaves, Notes on acts concerning," undated, box 28, file 23, Subseries D. Correspondence, Subject Files and Ledgers (Superintendent), 1791–1937, Eastern State Hospital, State Archives, Library of Virginia, Richmond.

69. "Committee Appointed on Asylums for Colored People, Report to the Association of Medical Superintendents for American Institutions for the Insane," box 29, file 43, Subseries D. Correspondence, Subject Files and Ledgers (Superintendent), 1791–1937, 1844, Eastern State Hospital Collection, State Library of Virginia, Richmond.

70. Recent scholarship casts a new light on free Blacks in the South. See Larry Koger, *Black Slaveowners: Free Black Slave Masters in South Carolina, 1790–1860* (Jefferson, NC: McFarland, 2010); and Jane G. Landers, ed., *Against the Odds: Free Blacks in the Slave Societies of the Americas* (New York: Routledge, 2013).

71. "Committee Appointed on Asylums for Colored People."

72. Wendy Gonaver's chapter about the 1840s and the Eastern Lunatic Asylum addresses the decisions of John Galt to open his asylum to the enslaved population. However, she does not mention the debates in the 1840s regarding the opening of a new institution that would be reserved only for black individuals. Gonaver, *Peculiar Institution*, 19–50.

73. "Committee Appointed on Asylums for Colored People."

74. McCandless, *Moonlight, Magnolias, and Madness*, 75–76.

75. On Galt and the abolitionist movement, see Gonaver, *Peculiar Institution*, 21; on Galt promoting interracial institutions, 28–35.

76. Ruth B. Caplan, *Psychiatry and the Community in Nineteenth-Century America: The Recurring Concern with the Environment in the Prevention and Treatment of Mental Illness* (New York: Basic Books, 1969), 60–61.

77. Christophe Prochasson and Anne Rasmussen, "Du bon usage de la dispute: Introduction," *Mil neuf cent: Revue d'histoire intellectuelle* 25, no. 1 (February 2007): 5–12. My translation.

78. On the construction of a public concern, see Elizabeth Sheppard, "Problème public," in *Dictionnaire des politiques publiques*, 3ᵉ edition (Paris: Presses de Sciences Po, 2010), 530–538.

2. The Strange Career of the 1840 Census Statistics

1. This chapter is based on Élodie Grossi, "Truth in Numbers? Emancipation, Race, and Federal Census Statistics in the Debates over Black Mental Health in the United States, 1840–1900," *Endeavour* 45, no. 1–2 (2021): 100766.

2. "Reflections on the Census of 1840," *Southern Literary Messenger* 9, no. 6 (1843): 341.

3. Edward Jarvis, "Statistics of Insanity in the United States," *Boston Medical and Surgical Journal* 27 (September 21, 1842): 119.

4. John Fulenwider Miller, "The Effects of Emancipation upon the Mental and Physical Health of the Negro of the South," *North Carolina Medical Journal* 38 (December 1896): 287–294.

5. Albert Deutsch, "The First U.S. Census of the Insane (1840) and Its Use as Pro-Slavery Propaganda," *Bulletin on the History of Medicine* 15 (January 1944): 469–482; Leon Litwack, *North of Slavery: The Negro in the Free States, 1790–1860* (Chicago: University of Chicago Press, 1961), 40–46; Theodore M. Porter, *The Rise of Statistical Thinking, 1820–1900* (Princeton, NJ: Princeton University Press, 1988), 37–38.

6. Margo Anderson and Stephen E. Fienberg, *Who Counts? The Politics of Census-Taking in Contemporary America* (New York: Russell Sage Foundation, 2001), 19.

7. Patricia Cline Cohen, *A Calculating People: The Spread of Numeracy in Early America* (Chicago: University of Chicago Press, 1988), 190; Paul Schor, *Counting Americans: How the U.S. Census Classified the Nation*, trans. Lys Ann Weiss (New York: Oxford University Press, 2017), 32–38. See also Melissa Nobles, *Shades of Citizenship: Race and the Census in Modern Politics* (Palo Alto, CA: Stanford University Press, 2000), 32.

8. In addition to the sources quoted previously, see Gerald N. Grob, "Edward Jarvis and the Federal Census," *Bulletin of the History of Medicine* 50 (Spring 1976): 4–27.

9. Jarvis, "Statistics of Insanity," 116–121.

10. See Gerald N. Grob, *Edward Jarvis and the Medical World of Nineteenth-Century America* (Knoxville: University of Tennessee Press, 1978); J. H. Cassedy, "Medical World of Madness, Morality, and Number," *Reviews in American History* 7 (June 1979): 219–223; and Grob, "Edward Jarvis and the Federal Census," 6.

11. Jarvis, "Statistics of Insanity," 119.

12. "Reflections on the Census of 1840," 340–352.

13. "Reflections on the Census of 1840," 351–352.

14. "Curious Statistical Facts," *Daily National Intelligencer*, June 15, 1843.

15. John C. Calhoun to Richard Pakenham, Senate Documents, 28 Cong., 1st sess., 50–53, April 18, 1844.

16. Richard Hofstadter, "From Calhoun to the Dixiecrats," *Social Research* 82, no. 1 (Spring 2015): 245–261.

17. Grossi, "Truth in Numbers?"

18. Stephen R. Haynes, *Noah's Curse: The Biblical Justification of American Slavery* (Oxford: Oxford University Press, 2002).

19. See Susan Branson, "Phrenology and the Science of Race in Antebellum America," *Early American Studies* 15, no. 1 (2017): 164–193; and James Poskett, "Phrenology, Correspondence, and the Global Politics of Reform, 1815–1848," *Historical Journal* 60 (2017): 409–442. On Morton, see Wendi A. Lindquist, "Stealing from the Dead: Scientists, Settlers, and Indian Burial Sites in Early-Nineteenth-Century Oregon," *Oregon Historical Quarterly* 115, no. 3 (Fall 2014): 324–343.

20. Lindquist, "Stealing from the Dead," 330.

21. John C. Calhoun, "Speech on the Reception of Abolition Petitions," February 6, 1837, in *The Works of John C. Calhoun*, vol. 2, ed. Richard Kenner Crallé (New York: D. Appleton, 1888), 626–627.

22. For example, see "Académie royale des Sciences. Séance du 17 décembre. Population des États-Unis, Statistique médicale," *Archives générales de médecine* 30 (1832): 574.

23. Ramón de la Sagra, "Statistique des aliénés et des sourds-muets dans les États-Unis de l'Amérique du Nord," *Annales médico-psychologiques* 1 (1843): 281–283. My translation.

24. James McCune Smith, "Freedom and Slavery for Afric-Americans (1844)," in *The Works of James McCune Smith: Black Intellectual and Abolitionist*, ed. John Stauffer (Oxford: Oxford University Press, 2006), 61–65.

25. "Meeting of 'Colored' Citizens of New York, New Jersey, Williamsburg, and Brooklyn, to Denounce John C. Calhoun and the Southern Slave Holders—Extraordinary Proceedings," *New York Herald*, May 6, 1844, 13.

26. Thomas C. Patterson, "An Archaeology of the History of Nineteenth-Century U.S. Anthropology: James McCune Smith, Radical Abolitionist and Anthropologist," *Journal of Anthropological Research* 69, no. 4 (2013): 459–484; William Seraile, "The Brief Diplomatic Career of Henry Highland Garnet," *Phylon* 46, no. 1 (1985): 71–81.

27. "Black Freedom," *Charleston Mercury* (September 30, 1851): 2.

28. David Correia, "Making Destiny Manifest: United States Territorial Expansion and the Dispossession of Two Mexican Property Claims in New Mexico, 1824–1899," *Journal of Historical Geography* 35, no. 1 (January 2009): 87–103.

29. Eric Foner, "The Wilmot Proviso Revisited," *Journal of American History* 56, no. 2 (September 1969): 262–279.

30. Marissa D. King and Heather A. Haveman, "Antislavery in America: The Press, the Pulpit, and the Rise of Antislavery Societies," *Administrative Science Quarterly* 53, no. 3 (September 2008): 492–528.

31. Carl Osthaus, *Partisans of the Southern Press: Editorial Spokesmen of the Nineteenth Century* (Lexington: University Press of Kentucky, 2014).

32. Stanford E. Chaillé, *A Memoir of the Insane Asylum of the State of Louisiana, at Jackson* (Baton Rouge: J. M. Taylor, 1858), 9.

33. William M. Overton, Charles Maurice Smith, and Beverley Tucker, "Slaves and Free Negroes," *Washington Sentinel*, September 1, 1854.

34. "Facts Worth Noticing," *Macon Weekly Telegraph*, November 4, 1856, 3.

35. L. Woodruff, "The Seventh United States Census," *Hunt's Merchants' Magazine and Commercial Review* 34 (1856): 172.

36. "Black and White Insanity," *Charleston Mercury*, April 24, 1857, 1.

37. James Freeman Clarke, "Condition of the Free Colored People of the United States," *Christian Examiner* 66, March 25, 1859, 246–265.

38. Robley Dunglison, "Dr. Dunglinson's Statistics of Insanity in the United States," *American Journal of Insanity* (1860).

39. Jonathan Earle and Diane Mutti Burke, eds., *Bleeding Kansas, Bleeding Missouri: The Long Civil War on the Border* (Topeka: University of Kansas Press, 2013).

40. Nicole Etcheson, "'Our lives, our fortunes and our sacred honors': The Kansas Civil War and the Revolutionary," *American Nineteenth Century History* 1, no. 1 (Spring 2000): 62–81.

41. Christopher Childers, *The Failure of Popular Sovereignty: Slavery, Manifest Destiny, and the Radicalization of Southern Politics* (Lawrence: University Press of Kansas, 2012).

42. "Statistics of Affliction," *Weekly Louisianian*, November 30, 1871, 4.

43. Joseph Jones, *General Medicine, Diseases of the Nervous System by Joseph Jones, M.D., Delivered Before the Louisiana State Medical Society at its 11th Annual Session, New Orleans, LA, April 1889* (New Orleans: L. Graham and Son, 1889), 19–20.

44. Stephen Cresswell, *Rednecks, Redeemers, and Race: Mississippi After Reconstruction, 1877–1917* (Jackson: University Press of Mississippi, 2006).

45. Shirley A. Hollis, "Neither Slave nor Free: The Ideology of Capitalism and the Failure of Radical Reform in the American South," *Critical Sociology* 35, no. 1 (2009): 9–27.

46. Jones, *General Medicine*, 21.

47. *Plaindealer*, May 16, 1890, 4.

48. "Freedom and the Negro," *The Conservative*, June 14, 1900: 4.

49. See Grace Elizabeth Hale, *Making Whiteness: The Culture of Segregation in the South, 1890–1940* (New York: Pantheon Books, 1998), 81. Hale quotes W. E. B. Du Bois, who wrote that southerners during Reconstruction represented themselves as "martyr[s] to inescapable fate." See Du Bois, *Black Reconstruction in America: An Essay Toward a History of the Part Which Black Folk Played in the Attempt to Reconstruct Democracy in America, 1860–1880* (New York: Harcourt, Brace and Company, 1935), 711–729; and A. A. Taylor, "Historians of the Reconstruction," *Journal of Negro History* 23 (January 1938): 16–34.

3. The Opening of Psychiatric Institutions for Black Patients in the South, 1860–1880

1. "Letter to Baldwin, Superintendent of Western Hospital, by Dr. Martin Scott," box 55, folder 24, Western State Hospital Collection, Library of Virginia. See also Élodie Grossi, "Médicaliser la folle Émancipation, soigner la folie noire? Le contexte d'ouverture du Central Lunatic State Asylum for Colored Insane en question," in *Imaginaire racial et oppositions identitaires (aire anglophone)*, ed. Michel Prum (Paris: L'Harmattan, 2016).

2. For a study on the memory of the war among the white southerners and the renewed vitality of the Lost Cause at the turn of the 1870s, see Benjamin G. Cloyd, *Haunted By Atrocity: Civil War Prisons in American Memory* (Baton Rouge: Louisiana State University Press, 2010).

3. See Aaron Sheehan-Dean, ed., *A Companion to the U.S. Civil War* (New York: John Wiley & Sons, 2014), 328–337.

4. This is an example of what Michel Foucault called the "problem of excess in speech" in his Collège de France course (1980–1981). Speech becomes prescription; verbalization processes strengthen it in a performative way and transform words into "truths." See also Mario Colucci, "Hystériques, internés, hommes infâmes: Michel Foucault et la résistance au pouvoir," *Sud/Nord* 1, no. 20 (2005): 123–145.

5. Bell I. Wiley, "Southern Reaction to Federal Invasion," *Journal of Southern History* 16, no. 4 (November 1950): 491–510; Stephen V. Ash, *When the Yankees Came: Conflict and Chaos in the Occupied South, 1861–1865* (Chapel Hill: University of North Carolina Press, 1995).

6. Robert W. Burg, "Amnesty, Civil Rights, and the Meaning of Liberal Republicanism, 1862–1872," *American Nineteenth Century History* 4, no. 3 (Fall 2003): 29–60.

7. See Stephen V. Ash, *A Massacre in Memphis: The Race Riot That Shook the Nation One Year After the Civil War* (New York: Hill and Wang, 2014); and Kevin R. Hardwick, "'Your Old Father Abe Lincoln Is Dead and Damned': Black Soldiers and the Memphis Race Riot of 1866," *Journal of Social History* 27, no. 1 (Autumn 1993): 109–128.

8. Altina L. Waller, "Community, Class and Race in the Memphis Riot of 1866," *Journal of Social History* 18, no. 2 (Winter 1984): 233–246.

9. Carolyn E. DeLatte, "The St. Landry Riot: A Forgotten Incident of Reconstruction Violence," *Louisiana History: The Journal of the Louisiana Historical Association* 17, no. 1 (Winter 1976): 41–49; Art Carden and Christopher J. Coyne, "The Political Economy of the Reconstruction Era's Race Riots," *Public Choice* 157, no. 1–2 (October 2013): 57–71; LeeAnna Keith, *The Colfax Massacre: The Untold Story of Black Power, White Terror, and the Death of Reconstruction* (New York: Oxford University Press, 2008).

10. I will use the notion of moral economy developed by E. P. Thompson to analyze the networks of values, affects, and rationalities in the South. See Thompson, "The Moral Economy of the English Crowd in the Eighteenth Century," *Past & Present* 50 (February 1971): 76–136.

11. All of these facilities changed their names over the course of the nineteenth century.

12. The Central Lunatic Asylum for Colored Insane changed its name at the turn of the twentieth century and became the Central State Hospital. I will use either name, depending on the historical period studied. See also Wendy Gonaver, *The Peculiar Institution and the Making of Modern Psychiatry, 1840–1880* (Chapel Hill: University of North Carolina Press, 2019), 173–193.

13. See Kirby Ann Randolph, "Central Lunatic Asylum for the Colored Insane: A History of African Americans with Mental Disabilities, 1844–1885" (PhD diss., University of Pennsylvania, 2003). See also Gonaver, *Peculiar Institution*, 181–193. Gonaver has recently written about the use of mechanical restraints on patients at the Central Lunatic Asylum, as well as how religion became a variable used by physicians to measure the degree of "excitement" of black patients, but not of Whites, when concluding that a patient needed to be restrained.

14. For a brief mention of this specific hospital in North Carolina, see Gonaver, *Peculiar Institution*, 191.

15. See A. H. Witmer, "Insanity in the Colored Race in the United States," *Alienist and Neurologist* 12 (1891): 19–30.

16. Whereas enslaved people constituted a minority of patients in the 1840s, their numbers increased drastically in the 1850s.

17. See Peter McCandless, *Moonlight, Magnolias, and Madness: Insanity in South Carolina from the Colonial Period to the Progressive Era* (Chapel Hill: University of North Carolina Press, 1996), 77.

18. Margot Minardi, *Making Slavery History: Abolitionism and the Politics of Memory in Massachusetts* (Oxford: Oxford University Press, 2010); Minardi, "Making Slavery Visible (Again): The Nineteenth-Century Roots of a Revisionist Recovery in New England," in *Politics of Memory: Making Slavery Visible in the Public Space,* ed. Ana Lucia Araujo (London: Routledge, 2012).

19. Joanne Pope Melish, *Disowning Slavery: Gradual Emancipation and "Race" in New England, 1780–1860* (Ithaca, NY: Cornell University Press, 1998).

20. Leon Litwack, *North of Slavery: The Negro in the Free States, 1790–1860* (Chicago: University of Chicago Press, 1961).

21. The Central Lunatic Asylum for the Colored Insane was first temporarily established in the walls of the former Howard's Grove Hospital, which in 1865 became an asylum under the direction of the Freedmen's Bureau. It was not until December 17, 1869, that it became the Virginia asylum by the action of General Canby (the military governor of Virginia under the occupation of the federal forces). When Governor Walker regained control of the state in 1870, the assembly voted for permanent incorporation of the asylum as a state institution. See "History of the Asylum," in *Report of the Board of Directors and Medical Superintendent of the Central Lunatic Asylum (for Colored Insane), Virginia, for the Year 1872–1873* (Richmond, VA: R. F. Walker, Superintendent of Public Printing, 1873), 16.

22. On the black institutions of the New South and of the Jim Crow era, see Edward L. Ayers, *The Promise of the New South: Life After Reconstruction* (Oxford: Oxford University Press, 1992); the classic work of C. Vann Woodward, *The Origins of the New South* (Baton Rouge: Louisiana State University Press, 1951); and Leon F. Litwack, *Trouble in Mind: Black Southerners in the Age of Jim Crow* (New York: Knopf, 1998), 271. Gretchen Long's book on the development of black institutions during Reconstruction, with the help of the Freedmen's Bureau, focuses on the efforts to defeat white medicine and treat black patients with fairness. Black patients developed resistance practices. See Long, *Doctoring Freedom: The Politics of African American Medical Care in Slavery and Emancipation* (Chapel Hill: University of North Carolina Press, 2012). On the management of hospitals for black patients during the transition period between slavery and freedom in the early 1860s, see Jim Downs, *Sick from Freedom: African American Illness and Suffering During the Civil War and Reconstruction* (Oxford: Oxford University Press, 2015).

23. Reference is made here to Michel Foucault's work on the generalization of psychiatric power and disciplinary technologies through the biopower system. Foucault's theory is extremely valuable, and the aim here is to focus more on the "positive" vision that the black elites of Virginia had of the institutions for black patients. See Foucault, *Le Pouvoir psychiatrique: Cours au Collège de France, 1973–1974* (Paris: Le Seuil, 2003); and Foucault, *Il faut défendre la société: Cours au Collège de France (1975–1976)* (Paris: Le Seuil, 1997). For social control in nineteenth-century asylums, see Pierangelo Di Vittorio, "De la psychiatrie à la biopolitique, ou la naissance de l'État bio-sécuritaire," in *Michel Foucault et le contrôle social*, ed. Alain Beaulieu (Laval: Presses de l'Université de Laval, 2005), 911–924.

24. Reconstruction was the period from 1865 to 1877, during which federal troops deployed in former Confederate states in order to establish the unity of federal power. During this short period, black patients from the South were able to gain citizenship, after the Fourteenth Amendment was ratified in 1868.

25. On the issue of education and segregation, see James Anderson, *The Education of Blacks in the South, 1860–1935* (Chapel Hill: University of North Carolina Press, 2010). On black legislators and their first votes, see Luther P. Jackson, *Negro Office-Holders in Virginia, 1865–1895* (Norfolk, VA: Guide Quality Press, 1945); Howard Rabinowitz, *Southern Black Leaders of the Reconstruction Era* (Urbana: University of Illinois Press, 1982); and Richard Lowe, *Republicans and Reconstruction in Virginia, 1856–70* (Charlottesville: University of Virginia Press, 1991).

26. See *Report of the Board of Directors* of 1871–1872, which lists the illnesses of the first patients of the hospital.

27. David Rothman, *The Discovery of the Asylum: Social Order and Disorder in the New Republic* (Boston: Little, Brown, 1971).

28. Michael B. Katz, *Poverty and Policy in American History* (New York: Academic Press, 1983), 6.

29. David Wagner, *The Poorhouse: America's Forgotten Institution* (New York: Rowman and Littlefield, 2005), 156.

30. Timothy Lockley, *Welfare and Charity in the Antebellum South* (Gainesville: University of Florida Press, 2007), 59.

31. "Act to permit for the Colored Insane of North Carolina," November 1874–March 1875, Senate Bills 771–829, North Carolina State Archives, Raleigh.

32. Motion, "Provided that No More Colored Insane Shall be Received in the Asylum at Raleigh," November 1874–March 1875, Senate Bills 771–829, North Carolina State Archives, Raleigh.

33. Cécile Vidal, ed., *Louisiana: Crossroads of the Atlantic World* (Philadelphia: University of Pennsylvania Press, 2014).

34. See, for example, "Rapport annuel de la Société Française de Bienfaisance et d'assistance mutuelle de la Nouvelle Orléans: hôpital français," box 1, file 2 (1843–1947), French Society of New Orleans Collection, Hill Memorial Library, Louisiana State University, Baton Rouge. I use the term *Creole* in the Louisiana sense, to refer to the black and white population born in the Americas, and often part of the social and cultural elite of the city of New Orleans, and not as synonymous with *white*.

35. John W. Blassingame, *Black New Orleans, 1860–1880* (Chicago: University of Chicago Press, 1973), 13.

36. Joseph Jones, *General Medicine, Diseases of the Nervous System by Joseph Jones, M.D., De-*

livered Before the Louisiana State Medical Society at its 11th Annual Session, New Orleans, LA, April 1889 (New Orleans: L. Graham and Son, 1889).

37. Christopher B. Bean, Too Great a Burden to Bear: The Struggle and Failure of the Freedmen's Bureau in Texas (New York: Fordham University Press, 2016), 144–145.

38. See John Duffy, The Rudolph Matas History of Medicine in Louisiana (Gretna: Pelican, 1976), 323–325.

39. "Letter from Governor Clyde R. Hoey to W. A. Dees, attorney at Law, Goldsboro, N.C," September 23, 1938, box 61, Hospitals, Orphanages, Training Schools, and Institutions, folder "State Hospital for the Insane, Goldsboro," Clyde R. Hoey, 1936–1941, Office of the Governor Collection, North Carolina State Archives, Raleigh.

40. "Letter from W. A. Dees to Governor Clyde R. Hoey, Raleigh, NC," September 28, 1938, box 61, Hospitals, Orphanages, Training Schools, and Institutions.

41. Leon C. Prieto and Simone T. A. Phipps, "Re-discovering Charles Clinton Spaulding's 'The Administration of Big Business': Insight into Early 20th Century African-American Management Thought," Journal of Management History 22, no. 1 (2016): 73–90.

42. "Letter from President Charles Clinton Spaulding, N.C. Mutual Life Insurance Co., Durham, NC to Governor Clyde R. Hoey, Durham, NC," June 21, 1940, box 61, Hospitals, Orphanages, Training Schools, and Institutions.

43. "Letter from the Governor Clyde R. Hoey, to President C. C. Spaulding, N.C. Mutual Life Insurance Co., Durham, NC," June 27, 1940, box 61, Hospitals, Orphanages, Training Schools, and Institutions.

44. Blassingame, Black New Orleans, 197.

45. "City Asylum," New Orleans Tribune, October 19, 1866; "City Asylum," New Orleans Times, July 21, 1871 (reprinted from the New York Herald, July 16, 1871). On informal segregation, see J. Curtis Waldo, Illustrated Visitor's Guide to New Orleans (New Orleans, LA: J. Curtis Waldo, 1879), 80; and Germaine A. Reed, "Race Legislation in Louisiana, 1864–1920," Louisiana History: The Journal of the Louisiana Historical Association 6, no. 4 (1965): 379–392.

46. "City Asylum," New Orleans Tribune, October 14, 1866.

47. See "Commemorative Calendar, Central Louisiana State Hospital, Centennial Celebration January 6, 1906–January 6, 2006," Louisiana and Lower Mississippi Valley Collections, LSU Libraries Special Collections, Hill Memorial Library, Louisiana State University, Baton Rouge.

48. Report of the Board of Administrators of the Louisiana Hospital for Insane of the State of Louisiana, to the Governor, Biennial Period Ending March 31st, 1908 (Baton Rouge: Daily State Publishing Co., 1908), 12–13.

49. See Carla Joinson, Vanished in Hiawatha: The Story of the Canton Asylum for Insane Indians (Lincoln: University of Nebraska Press, 2016).

50. Martin Summers, Madness in the City of Magnificent Intentions: A History of Race and Mental Illness in the Nation's Capital (New York: Oxford University Press, 2019), 41, 43.

51. Annual Report of the Central Louisiana State Hospital, 1941 to the Governor (Baton Rouge: State Printing Press, 1941), 109.

52. Plessy v. Ferguson, 163 U.S. 537 (1896), had the effect of permitting racial segregation on the principle of the separate but equal doctrine. Although the decision dates from 1896, local policies were already in place in the 1870s, particularly in Virginia.

53. "Anglo-Saxon Supremacy," *Semi-Weekly Messenger,* October 28, 1898, 2.

54. The white elite of the antebellum era had seen its political, social, and economic influence diminish after the defeat of the Confederate South. Black individuals' access to new civil rights after the ratification of the Thirteenth Amendment that abolished slavery, the Fourteenth Amendment that granted them the right to citizenship, and the Fifteenth Amendment that guaranteed their voting rights had been strongly criticized by Whites of the South, who were attached to their former privileges. On white women in the South who mobilized to restore the social order of the antebellum South during the Reconstruction era, see, for example, Jane Turner Censer, *The Reconstruction of White Southern Womanhood, 1865–1895* (Baton Rouge: Louisiana State University Press, 2003).

55. "Black Insanity," *Daily Press* (Newport, VA), January 17, 1906.

56. "Senator Patteson Proposes to Divide the School Funds—Would Benefit White Pupils," *Daily Press* (Newport, VA), January 17, 1906.

57. See Romain Huret, *La fin de la pauvreté ? Les experts sociaux et la Guerre contre la pauvreté aux États-Unis (1945–1974)* (Paris: EHESS, 2008); and Huret, *American Tax Resisters* (Cambridge, MA: Harvard University Press, 2014).

58. Lee J. Alston and Joseph P. Ferrie, *Southern Paternalism and the American Welfare State: Economics, Politics, and Institutions in the South, 1865–1965* (Cambridge: Cambridge University Press, 1999), 19.

59. John J. Donohue III, James J. Heckman, and Petra E. Todd, "The Schooling of Southern Blacks: The Roles of Legal Activism and Private Philanthropy, 1910–1960," *Quarterly Journal of Economics* 117, no. 1 (February 2002): 225, 228, and 236.

60. *Superintendent's Report of the Eastern NC Insane Asylum, also the Reports of the Chairman of the Directors and of the State Treasurer, for the Year of 1886* (Wilmington, NC: Messenger Steam Power Press Print, 1886), 9.

61. "City Asylum," *New Orleans Times,* July 21, 1871.

62. Joseph Jones, *General Medicine, Diseases of the Nervous System by Joseph Jones, M.D., Delivered Before the Louisiana State Medical Society at its 11th Annual Session, New Orleans, LA, April 1889* (New Orleans: L. Graham and Son, 1889), 66–68. Jones's essay about diagnoses is followed by remarks about various reports written by physicians on the cases of insanity, treatments, and financial situations of the public and private asylums in Louisiana.

63. "Commemorative Calendar."

64. Patients were sent to the asylum either by families or by the state.

65. *Forty-Fifth Annual Report of the Central State Hospital of Virginia (Petersburg) for the Fiscal Year Ending September 30, 1915* (Richmond: Davis Bottom, Superintendent of Public Printing, 1915), 23. For the use of the phrase "comfortably crowded," see *Report of the Board of Directors and Medical Superintendent of the Central Lunatic Asylum (for Colored Insane), Virginia, for the Year 1871–1872* (Richmond: R. F. Walker, Superintendent of Public Printing, 1872), 6.

66. *Fiftieth and Fifty-First Annual Reports of the Central State Hospital of Virginia (Petersburg) for the Fiscal Years Ending September 30, 1920 and 1921* (Richmond: Davis Bottom, Superintendent of Public Printing, 1921), 7.

67. *Forty-Ninth Annual Report of the Central State Hospital of Virginia (Petersburg) for the Fiscal Year Ending September 30, 1919* (Richmond: Davis Bottom, Superintendent of Public Printing,

1920), 19; *The One Hundred and Forty-Sixth Annual Report of the Eastern State Hospital of Virginia* (*at Williamsburg*) *for the Fiscal Year Ending September 30, 1919* (Richmond: Davis Bottom, Superintendent of Public Printing, 1919), 11.

68. See Gonaver, *Peculiar Institution*, 191–194.

69. On carceral institutions in the South, see Douglas A. Blackmon, *Slavery by Another Name: The Re-enslavement of Black Americans from the Civil War to World War II* (New York: Anchor, 2009); Davis M. Oshinsky, *Worse than Slavery: Parchman Farm and the Ordeal of Jim Crow Justice* (New York: The Free Press, 1996); and Talitha L. LeFlouria, *Chained in Silence: Black Women and Convict Labor in the New South* (Chapel Hill: University of North Carolina Press, 2015).

70. *Annual Report of the Board of Directors and the Superintendent of the Eastern North Carolina Insane Asylum, for the Year ending December 31, 1882.* Goldsboro, NC: Messenger Book and Job Printing House, 1883.

71. *Superintendent's Report of the Eastern NC Insane Asylum for the Year of 1884* (Goldsboro, NC: Messenger Steam Power Press Print, 1885), 8–9, 11–12.

72. *Superintendent's Report of the Eastern NC Insane Asylum, also the Reports of the Chairman of the Directors and of the State Treasurer, for the Year of 1886* (Wilmington, NC: Messenger Steam Power Press Print, 1886), 17.

73. *Superintendent's Report of the Eastern NC Insane Asylum, also the Reports of the Chairman of the Directors and of the State Treasurer, for the Year of 1889* (Wilmington, NC: Messenger Steam Power Press Print, 1889), 12.

74. See, for example, Robert Cassanello, *To Render Invisible: Jim Crow and Public Life in New South Jacksonville* (Gainesville: University of Florida Press, 2013). On recreational facilities, see Barbara C. Cruz, Michael J. Berson, and Donald Falls, "Swimming Not Allowed: Teaching About Segregated Public Beaches and Pools," *Social Studies* 103, no. 6 (November–December 2012): 252–259.

75. Andrew R. Highsmith and Ansley T. Erickson, "Segregation as Splitting, Segregation as Joining: Schools, Housing, and the Many Modes of Jim Crow," *American Journal of Education* 121, no. 4 (August 2015): 563–595.

76. For Florida black codes, see Joe M. Richardson, "Florida Black Codes," *Florida Historical Quarterly* 47, no. 4 (April 1969): 365–379.

77. See Luke Keele, William Cubbison, and Ismail White, "Suppressing Black Votes: A Historical Case Study of Voting Restrictions in Louisiana," *American Political Science Review* 115, no. 2 (March 2021): 694–700.

78. R. Volney Riser, "Disfranchisement, the U.S. Constitution, and the Federal Courts: Alabama's 1901 Constitutional Convention Debates the Grandfather Clause," *American Journal of Legal History* 48, no. 3 (July 2006): 237–279.

79. See, for example, Charles Vincent, *Black Legislators in Louisiana During Reconstruction* (Baton Rouge: Louisiana State University Press, 1976); Michael D. Cobb and Jeffery A. Jenkins, "Race and the Representation of Blacks' Interests During Reconstruction," *Political Research Quarterly* 54, no. 1 (March 2001): 181–204; and Chris W. Branam, "'The Africans Have Taken Arkansas': Political Activities of African Americans in the Reconstruction Legislature," *Arkansas Historical Quarterly* 73, no. 3 (Autumn 2014): 233–267.

80. Elaine Frantz Parsons, *Ku-Klux: The Birth of the Klan During Reconstruction* (Chapel Hill: University of North Carolina Press, 2015).

81. See Amy Louise Wood, "Lynching Photography and the Visual Reproduction of White Supremacy," *American Nineteenth Century History* 6, no. 3 (2005): 373–399.

82. Harvey Young, "The Black Body as Souvenir in American Lynching," *Theatre Journal* 57, no. 4 (December 2005): 639–657.

83. Equal Justice Initiative, *Lynching in America: Confronting the Legacy of Racial Terror,* 3rd ed. (Montgomery, AL: Equal Justice Initiative, 2017).

84. "State Board of Charities Calls Upon the People to Help the Insane," *Caucasian* 15, no. 2 (March 29, 1900): 1.

85. "Hospital for Colored Insane Very Crowded," *Public Welfare Progress* 4 (1923): 3, in Nell Battle Lewis Papers, North Carolina State Archives, Raleigh, box 2, file 1.

86. "Letter from W. C. Linville, M.D., to T. L. Gardner, Sheriff of Rockingham County, Reidsville, NC," July 18, 1929, box 7, file 1, "State Hospital for the Insane, Goldsboro Correspondence, 1929," General Correspondence, Institutions 1929–1932, Office of the Governor Collection, North Carolina State Archives, Raleigh.

87. Katherine Castles, "Quiet Eugenics: Sterilization in North Carolina's Institutions for the Mentally Retarded, 1945–1965," *Journal of Southern History* 68, no. 4 (November 2002): 850.

88. See Gregory N. Price, William Darity Jr., and Rhonda V. Sharpe, "Did North Carolina Economically Breed-Out Blacks During its Historical Eugenic Sterilization Campaign?" *American Review of Political Economy* 15, no. 1 (June 2020): 1.

89. Joanna Schoen, "Between Choice and Coercion: Women and the Politics of Sterilization in North Carolina, 1929–1975," *Journal of Women's History* 13, no. 1 (Spring 2001): 132.

90. Castles, "Quiet Eugenics," 855.

91. Angie C. Kennedy, "Eugenics, 'Degenerate Girls,' and Social Workers During the Progressive Era," *Affilia* 23, no. 1 (February 2008): 22–37.

92. Castles, "Quiet Eugenics," 862.

4. Race and Moral Treatment in Asylums and Hospitals in the South, 1870–1940

1. Joseph Jones, *General Medicine, Diseases of the Nervous System by Joseph Jones, M.D., delivered before the Louisiana State Medical Society at its 11th Annual Session, New Orleans, LA, April 1889* (New Orleans: L. Graham and Son, 1889), 19–21.

2. Jones, *General Medicine,* 21. See also R. Gregory Lande, *Madness, Malingering, and Malfeasance: The Transformation of Psychiatry and the Law in the Civil War Era* (Lincoln: Potomac Books, 2005), 157–192.

3. Lande, *Madness, Malingering, and Malfeasance,* 184.

4. Daniel Mason and Honor Hsin, "'A More Perfect Arrangement of Plants': The Botanical Model in Psychiatric Nosology, 1676 to the Present Day," *History of Psychiatry* 29, no. 2 (2018): 138. See also Abdullah Kraam, "Karl Ludwig Kahlbaum by Dr. Ewald Hecker (1899)," *History of Psychiatry* 19, no. 1 (2008): 77–80.

5. Marten W. DeVries et al., "Emil Kraepelin's Legacy: Systematic Clinical Observation and the Categorical Classification of Psychiatric Diseases," *European Archives of Psychiatry and Clinical Neuroscience* 258, suppl. 2 (2008): 1–2.

6. *Report of the Board of Directors and Medical Superintendent of the Central Lunatic Asylum (for Colored Insane), Virginia, for the Year 1871–1872* (Richmond: R. F. Walker, Superintendent of Public Printing, 1872).

7. Ann Clymer Bigelow, "Insanity in Civil War Ohio," *Ohio Valley History* 17, no. 2 (2017): 46–64.

8. *Report of the Board of Directors and Medical Superintendent of the Central Lunatic Asylum (for Colored Insane), Virginia, for the Year 1877–1878* (Richmond: R. F. Walker, Superintendent of Public Printing, 1878), 32.

9. *Report of the Board of Directors and Medical Superintendent of the Central Lunatic Asylum (for Colored Insane), Virginia, for the Year 1882–1883* (Richmond: R. F. Walker, Superintendent of Public Printing, 1883), 21.

10. *Report of the Board of Directors and Medical Superintendent of the Central Lunatic Asylum (for Colored Insane), Virginia, for the Year 1883–1884* (Richmond, Rush U. Deer, Superintendent of Public Printing, 1884), 26.

11. *Annual Report of the Central Lunatic Asylum of Virginia for the Fiscal Year 1886–1887* (Richmond: A. R. Micou, Superintendent of Public Printing, 1887), 35; *Annual Report of the Central Lunatic Asylum of the State of Virginia for the Fiscal Year Ending September 30, 1889* (Richmond: J. H. O'Bannon, Superintendent of Public Printing, 1889), 39.

12. *Annual Report of the Central Lunatic Asylum of the State of Virginia for the Fiscal Year Ending September 30, 1891* (Richmond: J. H. O'Bannon, Superintendent of Public Printing, 1891), 23. There were then 2,572 admissions that year.

13. *Annual Report of the Central Lunatic Asylum of the State of Virginia for the Fiscal Year Ending September 30, 1892* (Richmond: J. H. O'Bannon, Superintendent of Public Printing, 1892), 23.

14. *Annual Report of the Central State Hospital of the State of Virginia (Petersburg, VA.) for the Fiscal Year Ending September 30, 1895* (Richmond: J. H. O'Bannon, Superintendent of Public Printing, 1895), 21.

15. *Annual Report of the Central State Hospital of the State of Virginia (Petersburg, VA.) for the Fiscal Year Ending September 30, 1895* (Richmond: J. H. O'Bannon, Superintendent of Public Printing, 1895), 23. For the disappearance of these categories, see *Thirty-First Annual Report of the Central State Hospital of Virginia (Petersburg) for the Fiscal Year Ending September 30, 1901* (Richmond: J. H. O'Bannon: Superintendent of Public Printing, 1901), 27.

16. Gregory Claeys, "The 'Survival of the Fittest' and the Origins of Social Darwinism," *Journal of the History of Ideas* 61, no. 2 (April 2000): 223.

17. Michelle E. Martin, "Philosophical and Religious Influences on Social Welfare Policy in the United States: The Ongoing Effect of Reformed Theology and Social Darwinism on Attitudes Toward the Poor and Social Welfare Policy and Practice," *Journal of Social Work* 12, no. 1 (January 2012): 51–64, especially 55.

18. *Annual Report of the Central Lunatic Asylum of the State of Virginia for the Fiscal Year Ending September 30, 1889* (Richmond: J. H. O'Bannon, Superintendent of Public Printing, 1889), 43.

19. George M. Fredrickson, *The Black Image in the White Mind: The Debate on Afro-American Character and Destiny, 1817–1914* (New York: Harper & Row, 1971).

20. Nicolas Barreyre, "Réunifier l'Union: intégrer l'Ouest à la Reconstruction américaine, 1870–1872," *Revue d'Histoire Moderne et Contemporaine* 49, no. 4 (Autumn 2002): 7–36.

21. "The Chamber of Commerce Declares Against Negro Domination," *Semi-Weekly Messenger* (Wilmington, NC) (October 11, 1898): 3.

22. Eugene Genovese, *Roll, Jordan, Roll: The World the Slaves Made* (New York: Vintage, 1976), 399.

23. Joseph G. Tregle Jr., "Early New Orleans Society: A Reappraisal," *Journal of Southern History* 18 (February 1952): 34.

24. William H. Holcombe, "The Alternative: A Separate Nationality or the Africanization of the South," *Southern Literary Messenger* 32, no. 2 (February 1861): 81.

25. "Southern Medical and Surgical Journal," box 3, file 66–68, Joseph Jones Papers (Manuscripts, 1866–1876), Mss. no. 468, Louisiana and Lower Mississippi Valley Collections, LSU Libraries Special Collections, Louisiana State University, Baton Rouge.

26. "Confederate States Medical and Surgical Journal," box 3, file 66–68; and "Southern Historical Society," file 69–70, box 3, in Joseph Jones Papers, (Manuscripts, 1866–1876).

27. Stanford Emerson Chaillé, "Vital Statistics Applied to the Military-Reconstruction Politics of Louisiana," *New Orleans Medical and Surgical Journal* (1875): 20; Chaillé, "Intimidation and the Number of White and of Colored Voters in Louisiana in 1876," *New Orleans Medical and Surgical Journal* (1876).

28. Andrew Abbott, *A System of Professions: An Essay on the Division of Expert Labor* (Chicago: University of Chicago Press, 1988). For an application of Abbott's theory, see Pam Grossman, "Responding to Our Critics: From Crisis to Opportunity in Research on Teacher Education," *Journal of Teacher Education* 59, no. 1 (January 2008): 11.

29. Gil Eyal, "For a Sociology of Expertise: The Social Origins of the Autism Epidemic," *American Journal of Sociology* 118, no. 4 (January 2013): 863–907.

30. See Elsa Dorlin, *La matrice de la race: Généalogie sexuelle et coloniale de la Nation française* (Paris: La Découverte, 2008); and Paul Chodoff, "Hysteria and Women," *American Journal of Psychiatry* 139, no. 5 (1982): 545–551.

31. Theodore Diller, "Causes of Insanity," *Pittsburgh Medical Review* 5 (October 1891): 295–296.

32. Maxime Du Camp, *Les Convulsions de Paris* (Paris: Librairie Hachette, 1878), ii, 131, and 470–471. All translations are my own.

33. "Immigration and Insanity," in *Reports of the Immigration Commission*, vol. 2 (Washington, DC: Government Printing Office, 1910), 227.

34. See John Radzilowski, "Fecund Newcomers or Dying Ethnics? Demographic Approaches to the History of Polish and Italian Immigrants and Their Children in the United States, 1880 to 1980," *Journal of American Ethnic History* 27, no. 1 (Fall 2007): 68.

35. On the Irish famine, see Susan Campbell Bartoletti, *Black Potatoes: The Story of the Great Irish Famine, 1845–1850* (Boston: Houghton Mifflin Harcourt, 2014).

36. "Immigration and Insanity," 236, 246, 250–251.

37. Judson B. Andrews, "The Distribution and Care of the Insane in the United States," *American Journal of Insanity* 44, no. 2 (1887): 194.

38. *Superintendent's Report of the Eastern NC Insane Asylum, also the Report of the Treasurer, for the Year of 1890* (Wilmington: Messenger Steam Power Presses, 1890), 6.

39. For classic books about the Great Migration, see Arnold Hirsch, *Making the Second Ghetto* (Chicago: University of Chicago Press, 1998); and James Grossman, *Land of Hope: Chicago, Black Southerners, and the Great Migration* (Chicago: University of Chicago Press, 1989).

40. Diller, "Causes of Insanity," 294. See also A. H. Witmer, "Insanity in the Colored Race in the United States," *Alienist and Neurologist* 12 (1891): 19–30.

41. "Statistics of Affliction," *Weekly Louisianian* (November 30, 1871): 4.

42. Hodges, J. Addison, "The Effect of Freedom upon the Physical and Psychological Development of the Negro," *Virginia Medical Semi-Monthly* 5 (May 1900): 106–110.

43. Gerald Grob, *Mental Illness and American Society, 1875–1940* (Princeton, NJ: Princeton University Press, 1987), 25.

44. *Report of the Board of Directors and Medical Superintendent of the Central Lunatic Asylum (for Colored Insane), Virginia, for the Year 1871–1872* (Richmond: R. F. Walker, Superintendent of Public Printing, 1872), 25.

45. Stanford Emerson Chaillé, *A Memoir of the Insane Asylum of the State of Louisiana, at Jackson* (Baton Rouge, LA: J. M. Taylor, 1858), 7.

46. Jack T. Kirby, "Black and White in the Rural South, 1915–1954," *Agricultural History* 58, no. 3 (July 1984): 411.

47. Daniel B. Novak, *The Wheel of Servitude: Black Forced Labor After Slavery* (Lexington: University Press of Kentucky, 1978).

48. Alex Lichtenstein, *Twice the Work of Free Labor: The Political Economy of Convict Labor in the New South* (London: Verso, 1996), xvii.

49. Douglas A. Blackmon, *Slavery by Another Name: The Re-enslavement of Black Americans from the Civil War to World War II* (New York: Anchor, 2009).

50. David M. Oshinsky, *Worse than Slavery: Parchman Farm and the Ordeal of Jim Crow Justice* (New York: The Free Press, 1996).

51. Talitha L. LeFlouria, *Chained in Silence: Black Women and Convict Labor in the New South* (Chapel Hill: University of North Carolina Press, 2015), 107–108.

52. Other publications have shown the extent to which work was a therapeutic order that organized most asylums in the United States; see, for example, Grob, *Mental Illness and American Society*, 23.

53. Philippe Pinel is seen today as one of the first and most influential French pioneers of psychiatry. At the beginning of the nineteenth century, he organized a major reform of the treatment institutions by medicalizing the care of the sick and suppressing corporal punishment against them. See James Harris, "Pinel Orders the Chains Removed From the Insane at Bicêtre," *Archives of General Psychiatry* 60, no. 5 (2003): 442.

54. Philippe Pinel, *Traité médico-philosophique sur l'aliénation mentale, Seconde édition, entièrement refondue et très-augmentée* (Paris: J. Ant. Brosson, 1809), 240. My translation. On the bad English translation of the first edition of the treatise published in 1806, see Dora B. Weiner, "Betrayal! The 1806 English Translation of Pinel's traité médico-philosophique sur l'aliénation mentale ou la manie," *Gesnerus* 57 (2000): 42–50.

55. Committee Appointed on Asylums for Colored People, "Report to the Association of Medical Superintendents for American Institutions for the Insane," 1844, Superintendent Files, box 29, file 43, Eastern State Hospital Collection, Library of Virginia, Richmond.

56. On polygenism, see Terence D. Keel, "Religion, Polygenism and the Early Science of Human Origins," *History of the Human Sciences* 26, no. 2 (April 2013): 4, 16, and 28.

57. "Southern Medical Reports," *De Bow's Review* 9, no. 3 (September 1850): 296.

58. "History of Institutions Shows a Growth of Ideas," *Public Welfare Progress* (1923): 5, in Nell Battle Lewis Papers, North Carolina State Archives, Raleigh, box 2, file 1.

59. Grace Elizabeth Hale, *Making Whiteness: The Culture of Segregation in the South, 1890–1940* (New York: Pantheon, 1998).

60. On black women leaders, see Glenda Gilmore, *Gender and Jim Crow: Women and the Politics of White Supremacy in North Carolina, 1896–1920* (Chapel Hill: University of North Carolina Press, 1996).

61. Linda Gordon, *The Second Coming of the KKK: The Ku Klux Klan of the 1920s and the American Political Tradition* (New York: Liveright, 2017). On southern political culture in the 1920s, see also Anne Stefani, *Unlikely Dissenters: White Southern Women in the Fight for Racial Justice, 1920–1970* (Gainesville: University Press of Florida, 2015).

62. See David Cecelski, *Along Freedom Road: Hyde County, North Carolina, and the Fate of Black Schools in the South* (Chapel Hill: University of North Carolina Press, 1994).

63. Hugh M. Browne, "Method of Education and Teaching for the Children of Undeveloped Races," *Southern Workman and Hampton School Record: 1899* (Hampton, VA: Hampton Normal and Agricultural Institute, 1899): 483–487.

64. *Report of the Board of Directors and Medical Superintendent of the Central Lunatic Asylum (for Colored Insane), Virginia, for the Year 1871–1872* (Richmond: R. F. Walker, Superintendent of Public Printing, 1872), 8.

65. *Superintendent's Report of the Eastern NC Insane Asylum, also the Reports of the Chairman of the Directors and of the State Treasurer for the Year of 1886* (Wilmington, NC: Messenger Steam Power Press Print, 1886), 16–17.

66. Nell Battle Lewis, "Daily Routine," box 1, file 1, Nell Battle Lewis Papers, North Carolina State Archives, Raleigh.

67. "November 5, 1920," box 551, file 1 (Dorothea Dix Hospital; Cherry Hospital, Institution, Mental; Miscellanea, 1920), Office of the Governor Collection, North Carolina State Archives, Raleigh.

68. William J. Drewry, "Care and Condition of the Insane in Virginia," in *Proceedings of the National Conference of Charities and Correction,* ed. Alexander Johnson (Fort Wayne: Press of Fort Wayne Printing, 1908), 312.

69. On slavery and capitalism, see Sven Beckert and Seth Rickman, eds., *Slavery's Capitalism: A New History of American Economic Development* (Philadelphia: University of Pennsylvania Press, 2016); Walter Johnson, *River of Dark Dreams: Slavery and Empire in the Cotton Kingdom* (Cambridge, MA: Harvard University Press, 2013); Edward Baptist, *The Half Has Never Been Told: Slavery and the Making of American Capitalism* (London: Hachette, 2016); Sven Beckert, *Empire of Cotton: A Global History* (New York: Knopf Doubleday, 2014); and Eric Williams, *Capitalism and Slavery* (Chapel Hill: University of North Carolina Press, 1994). For a substantial revision of Sven Beckert's thesis, see Alan L. Olmstead and Paul W. Rhode, "Cotton, Slavery, and the New History of Capitalism," *Explorations in Economic History* 67 (January 2018): 1–17. The work of black patients in southern psychiatric institutions is a continuation of the relationship

between slavery and capitalism in that it presents the same mode of economic exploitation of black labor during a later period. The methods of this exploitation are of course different, the medical power also coming into the balance.

70. Yann Moulier Boutang, *De l'esclavage au salariat: économie historique du salariat bridé* (Paris: Presses Universitaires de France, 1998).

71. *Report of the Board of Directors and Medical Superintendent of the Central Lunatic Asylum (for Colored Insane), Virginia, for the Year 1872–1873* (Richmond: R. F. Walker, Superintendent of Public Printing, 1873), 44.

72. James Lawrence Thompson, *Shattered Minds: Fifty Years at the South Carolina State Hospital for the Insane* (Columbia: South Carolina Department of Mental Health, 1989), 7.

73. Oshinsky, *Worse Than Slavery;* Lichtenstein, *Twice the Work of Free Labor;* Matthew J. Mancini, *One Dies, Get Another: Convict Leasing in the American South, 1866–1928* (Columbia: University of South Carolina Press, 1996); Mancini, "Race, Economics, and the Abandonment of Convict Leasing," *Journal of Negro History* 63, no. 4 (1978): 339–340.

74. *Superintendent's Report of the Eastern NC Insane Asylum for the Year of 1884* (Goldsboro, NC: Messenger Steam Power Press Print, 1885), 9.

75. *Superintendent's Report of the Eastern NC Insane Asylum, also the Reports of the Chairman of the Directors and of the State Treasurer, for the Year of 1886* (Wilmington, NC: Messenger Steam Power Press Print, 1886), 15.

76. *Superintendent's Report of the Eastern NC Insane Asylum, also the Report of the Treasurer, for the Year of 1890* (Wilmington, NC: Messenger Steam Power Print, 1890), 19.

77. *Report of the Board of the Administrators of the Central Louisiana State Hospital at Pineville, To his Excellency, the Governor, Biennial Period Ending March 31, 1934* (Alexandria: Standard Printing Co., Inc., 1934).

78. Matthew Fox-Amato, *Exposing Slavery: Photography, Human Bondage, and the Birth of Modern Visual Politics in America* (Oxford: Oxford University Press, 2019), 70.

79. *Report of the Board of Administrators of the Louisiana Hospital for Insane of the State of Louisiana, to the Governor, Biennial Period Ending March 31st, 1908* (Baton Rouge: Daily State Publishing Co., 1908), 23.

80. *Report of the Board of Directors and Medical Superintendent of the Central Lunatic Asylum (for Colored Insane), Virginia, for the Year 1871–1872* (Richmond: R. F. Walker, Superintendent of Public Printing, 1872), 7.

81. Michel Foucault, *Le Pouvoir psychiatrique: Cours au Collège de France, 1973–1974* (Paris: Le Seuil, 2003), 138. My translation.

82. Mario Colucci, "Hystériques, internés, hommes infâmes: Michel Foucault et la résistance au pouvoir," *Sud/Nord* 1, no. 20 (2005): 123–145.

83. Judith N. Shklar, *American Citizenship: The Quest for Inclusion* (Cambridge, MA: Harvard University Press, 1991).

84. Case 1885: mental examination (January 31, 1911), Elizabeth Hospital Archives, National Archives and Records Administration (NARA), Record Group (RG) 418, Entry 66, Washington, DC. Quoted in Matthew Gambino, "'These strangers within our gates': Race, Psychiatry and Mental Illness Among Black Americans at St. Elizabeths Hospital in Washington, DC, 1900–40," *History of Psychiatry* 19, no. 4 (December 2008): 405.

85. Michel Foucault, *Il faut défendre la société: Cours au Collège de France, 1975–1976* (Paris: Le Seuil, 1997), 8–9. My translation.

86. *Superintendent's Report of the Eastern NC Insane Asylum for the Year of 1884* (Goldsboro, NC: Messenger Steam Power Press Print, 1885), 13.

87. "State Hospital at Goldsboro, NC," box 551, file 1, Office of the Governor Collection.

88. Blackmon, *Slavery by Another Name*.

5. The Fabric of Epidemiological Otherness and Pathological Bodies, 1880–1940

1. See Martin Summers, *Madness in the City of Magnificent Intentions: A History of Race and Mental Illness in the Nation's Capital* (New York: Oxford University Press, 2019), 145, 148–149.

2. For the history of psychoanalysis in the United States in the following decades, particularly during the heyday of its public impact from the 1950s through the 1970s, see Mitchell G. Ash, "Americanizing Psychoanalysis," *Modern Intellectual History* 14, no. 2 (August 2017): 607–617.

3. Carl Jung, "Letter from Doctor Jung," *Psychoanalytic Review* 1, no. 1 (November 1913): 117–118.

4. Smith Ely Jeliffe and William Alanson White, *Diseases of the Nervous System: A Text-Book of Neurology and Psychiatry* (Philadelphia: Lea and Febinger, 1915); William Alanson White, *Mental Mechanisms* (New York: Journal of Nervous and Mental Disease Publishing, 1911); White, *Outlines of Psychiatry* (New York: Journal of Nervous and Mental Disease Publishing, 1911); White, *Thoughts of a Psychiatrist on the War and After* (New York: P. B. Hoeber, 1919).

5. Karl Abraham, *Dreams and Myths: A Study in Race Psychology*, trans. William A. White (New York: Journal of Nervous and Mental Disease Publishing, 1913), 72.

6. Historians such as Matthew Gambino and Martin Summers have delivered insightful analyses of the treatments of black patients at the St. Elizabeths hospital. See Matthew Gambino, "'These strangers within our gates': Race, Psychiatry and Mental Illness Among Black Americans at St. Elizabeths Hospital in Washington, DC, 1900–40," *History of Psychiatry* 19 (2008): 387–408; and Summers, *Madness*.

7. *Report of the Board of Administrators of the Louisiana Hospital for Insane of the State of Louisiana, to the Governor, Biennial Period Ending March 31st, 1908* (Baton Rouge: Daily State Publishing Co., 1908), 12–28.

8. *Thirty-Fourth Annual Report of the Central State Hospital of Virginia (Petersburg) for the Fiscal Year Ending September 30, 1904 and Historical Sketch of Hospital* (Richmond: J. H. O'Bannon: Superintendent of Public Printing, 1904), 10; and *Thirty-Sixth Annual Report of the Central State Hospital of Virginia (Petersburg) for the Fiscal Year Ending September 30, 1906* (Richmond: Davis Bottom: Superintendent of Public Printing, 1906), 11.

9. David Healy, *The Antidepressant Era* (Cambridge, MA: Harvard University Press, 1997), 13. See also Paul Hoff, "The Kraepelinian Tradition," *Dialogues in Clinical Neuroscience* 17, no. 1 (2005): 31–41; and Talya Greene, "The Kraepelinian Dichotomy: The Twin Pillars Crumbling?," *History of Psychiatry* 18, no. 3 (2007): 361–379.

10. Gerald Grob, *The Inner World of American Psychiatry, 1890–1940* (New Brunswick, NJ: Rutgers University Press, 1985), 8.

11. Constance McGovern, *Masters of Madness: Social Origins of the American Psychiatric Profession* (Burlington: University of Vermont Press, 1985), 158.

12. E. M. Green, "Psychoses Among Negroes—A Comparative Study," *Journal of Nervous and Mental Disease* 41, no. 11 (1914): 697–708. See also Green, "Manic-Depressive Psychosis in the Negro," *American Journal of Insanity* 73 (1917): 619–626.

13. Dennis Doyle, *Psychiatry and Racial Liberalism in Harlem, 1936–1968* (Rochester, NY: University of Rochester Press, 2016), 21.

14. See Laura D. Hirshbein, "Science, Gender, and the Emergence of Depression in American Psychiatry, 1952–1980," *Journal of the History of Medicine and Allied Sciences* 61, no. 2 (2006): 223.

15. Arrah B. Evarts, "Dementia Praecox in the Colored Race," *Psychoanalytic Review* 1, no. 4 (October 1914), 396.

16. *Superintendent's Report of the Eastern NC Insane Asylum, also the Reports of the Chairman of the Directors and of the State Treasurer, for the Year of 1889* (Wilmington, NC: Messenger Steam Power Press Print, 1889), 14–15, 40.

17. On these stereotypes, see Angela Y. Davis, *Women, Race & Class* (New York: Vintage, 1983); and Ayumu Kaneko, "The Politics of the Black Rapist Myth: American Racial Violence, Gender and Class at the Turn of the 20th Century," *J-Stage* 3 (2007): 5–18.

18. Davis, *Women, Race & Class*, 176.

19. Diane Miller Sommerville, *Rape and Race in the Nineteenth-Century South* (Chapel Hill: University of North Carolina Press, 2004).

20. On lynchings, see Stewart E. Tolnay and E. M. Beck, *A Festival of Violence: An Analysis of Southern Lynchings, 1882–1930* (Urbana: University of Illinois Press, 1992); Herbert Shapiro, *White Violence and Black Response: From Reconstruction to Montgomery* (Amherst: University of Massachusetts Press, 1988); Martha Hodes, *White Women, Black Men: Illicit Sex in the Nineteenth-Century South* (New Haven, CT: Yale University Press, 1997); Trudier Harris, *Exorcising Blackness: Historical and Literary Lynching and Burning Rituals* (Bloomington: Indiana University Press, 1984); Terence Finnegan, "Lynching and Political Power in Mississippi and South Carolina," in *Under Sentence of Death: Lynching in the South*, ed. W. Fitzhugh Brundage (Chapel Hill: University of North Carolina Press, 1997), 189–218; and W. Fitzhugh Brundage, *Lynching in the New South: Georgia and Virginia, 1880–1930* (Urbana: University of Illinois Press, 1993).

21. Laura Edwards, "Captives of Wilmington: The Riot and Historical Memories of Political Conflict, 1865–1898," in *Democracy Betrayed: The Wilmington Race Riot of 1898 and Its Legacy*, ed. David S. Cecelski and Timothy B. Tyson (Chapel Hill: University of North Carolina Press, 2000), 108, 112.

22. On Thomas Dixon, see George M. Fredrickson, *The Black Image in the White Mind: The Debate on Afro-American Character and Destiny, 1817–1914* (New York: Harper & Row, 1971), 280.

23. Lee D. Baker, *From Savage to Negro: Anthropology and the Construction of Race, 1896–1954* (Berkeley: University of California Press, 1998).

24. Stephen Kantrowitz, *Ben Tillman and the Reconstruction of White Supremacy* (Chapel Hill: University of North Carolina Press, 2000), 165.

25. See James F. Davis, *Who Is Black? One Nation's Definition* (University Park: Pennsylvania State University Press, 2001). On the hypodescent rule in the state of Virginia, for example, see

Joshua D. Rothman, *Notorious in the Neighborhood: Sex and Families Across the Color Line in Virginia, 1787–1861* (Chapel Hill: University of North Carolina Press, 2003), 68.

26. See Paul Schor, "The Disappearance of the 'Mulatto' as the End of Inquiry into the Composition of the Black Population of the United States," in *Counting Americans: How the U.S. Census Classified the Nation*, trans. Lys Ann Weiss (New York: Oxford University Press, 2017), 155–168.

27. See Henry Havelock Ellis, "Sexual Inversion in Women," *Alienist and Neurologist* 16 (1895): 143–144.

28. On Bevis, see Summers, *Madness*, 142–146.

29. William V. Bevis, "Psychological Traits of the Southern Negro with Observations as to Some of His Psychoses," *American Journal of Psychiatry* 78 (1921–1922): 70.

30. Evarts, "Dementia Praecox in the Colored Race," 397.

31. Winthrop D. Jordan, "Historical Origins of the One-Drop Racial Rule in the United States," *Journal of Critical Mixed Race Studies* 1, no. 1 (2014): 112–114.

32. Thelma Jennings, "'Us Colored Women Had to Go Though a Plenty': Sexual Exploitation of African-American Slave Women," *Journal of Women's History* 1, no. 3 (1990): 45–74. As Jennings explains, "When it was profitable to exploit women as if they were men in the work force, slaveholders regarded female slaves as genderless. But when they could be exploited in ways designed only for women, they were exclusively female—subordinate and unequal to all men." In this masterful article, Jennings reveals that white patriarchs often subjected enslaved females to forced reproduction through rape to increase the number of enslaved people on their land and therefore their profits.

33. See Pauli Murray, ed., *States' Laws on Race and Color* (Athens: University of Georgia Press, 1997).

34. See Schor, "Disappearance of the 'Mulatto,'" 155–168.

35. See Charles S. Bryan, *Asylum Doctor: James Woods Babcock and the Red Plague of Pellagra* (Columbia: University of South Carolina Press, 2014).

36. W. C. Linville, "Letter to Chas. O'H. Laughinghouse," October 10, 1929, box 7, file 1 (Goldsboro Records), General Correspondence, Institutions 1929–1932, Office of the Governor Collection, North Carolina State Archives, Raleigh.

37. Chas. O'H. Laughinghouse, "Letter of October 11, 1929," box 7, file 1 (Goldsboro Records), Office of the Governor Collection.

38. See A. H. Witmer, "Insanity in the Colored Race in the United States," *Alienist and Neurologist* 12 (1891): 19.

39. *Superintendent's Report of the Eastern NC Insane Asylum for the Year of 1884* (Goldsboro, NC: Messenger Steam Power Press Print, 1885), 12.

40. Martin Summers, "Suitable Care of the African When Afflicted with Insanity: Race, Madness, and Social Order in Comparative Perspective," *Bulletin of the History of Medicine* 84, no. 1 (Spring 2010): 58–91.

41. *Report of the Eastern NC Insane Asylum for the Year of 1883* (Goldsboro, NC: Messenger Steam Power Press Print, 1884), 15.

42. Summers, "Suitable Care," 78; Charles Prudhomme, "The Problem of Suicide in the American Negro," *Psychoanalytic Review* 25 (1938): 187–204, especially 194.

43. On psychoanalysis and the theories on civilization, see Summers, "Suitable Care," 79.

44. On culture and biology, see Summers, "Suitable Care," 70–74.

45. J. D. Roberts, "Insanity in the Colored Race," in *Report of the Eastern NC Insane Asylum for the Year of 1883, Goldsboro, NC* (Goldsboro, NC: Messenger Steam Power Print, 1884), 120.

46. See Matthew Gambino, "'The Savage Heart Beneath the Civilized Exterior': Race, Citizenship, and Mental Illness in Washington, DC, 1900–1940," *Disability Studies Quarterly* 28, no. 3 (Summer 2008); and Gambino, "Fevered Decisions: Race, Ethics, and Clinical Vulnerability in the Malarial Treatment of Neurosyphilis, 1922–1953," *Hastings Center Report* 45, no. 4 (July–August 2015): 39–50.

47. Grob, *Inner World of American Psychiatry,* 9.

48. Arrah B. Evarts, "The Ontogenetic Against the Phylogenetic Elements in the Psychoses of the Colored Race," *Psychoanalytic Review* 3 (1916): 272. See also Anne C. Rose, *Psychology and Selfhood in the Segregated South* (Chapel Hill: University of North Carolina Press, 2009), 193.

49. Summers, *Madness,* 146.

50. John E. Lind, "The Dream as a Simple Wish-Fulfillment in the Negro," *Psychoanalytic Review* 1, no. 3 (1913): 300. This quote is also discussed by Summers, though he does not note the same paradox between the pursuit of universalist science and the separation of treatments for Blacks and Whites. See Summers, *Madness,* 149.

51. Sander L. Gilman focuses on the way in which Freud's writings dealt indirectly with images of racial difference and how the latter shaped the questions of psychoanalysis, especially regarding gender. The book focuses on Jewish identity and its portrayal as the "racial other" in the early twentieth century context of anti-Semitism in Europe but does not deal with blackness. See Gilman, *Freud, Race, and Gender* (Princeton, NJ: Princeton University Press, 1995).

52. Todd Savitt, "The Use of Blacks for Medical Experimentation and Demonstration in the Old South," *Journal of Southern History* 48, no. 3 (1982): 331–348; Deirdre Cooper Owens, *Medical Bondage: Race, Gender, and the Origins of American Gynecology* (Athens: University of Georgia Press, 2017); Daina Ramey Berry, *The Price for Their Pound of Flesh: The Value of the Enslaved, from Womb to Grave, in the Building of a Nation* (Boston: Beacon Press, 2017).

53. John E. Lind, "Diagnostic Pitfalls in the Examinations of Negroes," *New York Medical Journal* 99, no. 26 (1914): 1286–1287.

54. John E. Lind, "The Color Complex in the Negro," *Psychoanalytic Review* 1, no. 4 (October 1914): 404–405.

55. Alfred Adler, *Über den nervosen Character* (Göttingen: Vandenhoeck & Ruprecht, 1912); Sigmund Freud, *Die Traumdeutung,* 7th ed. (Leipzig: Franz Deuticke, 1924), quoted in Lind, "Color Complex."

56. Lind, "Color Complex," 404–405.

57. On other publications by Mary O'Malley, see Summers, *Madness,* 142–149, 164–166, 184, 193, 213, and 256.

58. See Grob, *Inner World of American Psychiatry,* 9.

59. Andrew Scull, "From Madness to Mental Illness: Medical Men as Moral Entrepreneurs," *European Journal of Sociology* 16, no. 2 (1975): 218–251. See also Eliot Freidson, *Profession of Medicine: A Study of the Sociology of Applied Knowledge* (Chicago: University of Chicago Press, 1970).

Epilogue: An Everlasting Story:
Race and Psychiatry in the United States Today

1. The international symposium "Medicine and Healing in the Age of Slavery," held at Rice University, coincidentally marked the thirtieth anniversary of Todd Savitt's book.

2. See Ronald Littlewood, "Psychiatric Diagnosis and Racial Bias: Empirical and Interpretative Approaches," *Social Science & Medicine* 34, no. 2 (January 1992): 141–149; Thomas W. Pavkov, Dan A. Lewis, and John S. Lyons, "Psychiatric Diagnoses and Racial Bias: An Empirical Investigation," *Professional Psychology: Research and Practice* 20, no. 6 (December 1989): 364–368; Marti Loring and Brian Powell, "Gender, Race, and DSM-III: A Study of the Objectivity of Psychiatric Diagnostic Behavior," *Journal of Health and Social Behavior* 29, no. 1 (March 1988): 1–22; Arthur L. Whaley, "Ethnicity/Race, Paranoia, and Psychiatric Diagnoses: Clinician Bias Versus Sociocultural Differences," *Journal of Psychopathology and Behavioral Assessment* 19, no. 1 (March 1997): 1–20; William B. Lawson, Nancy Hepler, and Jack Holladay, "Race as a Factor in Inpatient and Outpatient Admissions and Diagnosis," *Psychiatric Services* 45, no. 1 (April 1994): 72–74; and Glyn Lewis, Caroline Croft-Jeffreys, and Anthony David, "Are British Psychiatrists Racist?" *British Journal of Psychiatry* 157, no. 3 (September 1990): 410–415.

3. Mical Raz, *What's Wrong with the Poor? Psychiatry, Race, and the War on Poverty* (Chapel Hill: University of North Carolina Press, 2013); Helena Hansen, Philippe Bourgois, and Ernest Drucker, "Pathologizing Poverty: New Forms of Diagnosis, Disability, and Structural Stigma Under Welfare Reform," *Social Science & Medicine* 103 (February 2014): 76–83.

4. See Colin Samson, "Inequality, the New Right and Mental Health Care Delivery in the United States in the Reagan Era," *Critical Social Policy* 10, no. 29 (October 1990): 40–57; Anastasia Cooper, "The Ongoing Correctional Chaos in Criminalizing Mental Illness: The Realignment's Effects on California Jails," *Hastings Women's Law Journal* 24, no. 2 (2013): 339–361; and Marian Moser Jones, "Creating a Science of Homelessness During the Reagan Era," *Milbank Quarterly* 93, no. 1 (March 2015): 139–178. See also Loïc Wacquant, "Deadly Symbiosis: When Ghetto and Prison Meet and Mesh," *Punishment & Society* 3, no. 1 (January 1, 2001): 95–133.

Bibliography

Newspapers and Magazines

The Caucasian (Raleigh, NC)
Charleston Mercury (South Carolina)
Daily National Intelligencer (Washington, DC)
Daily Press (Newport, VA)
Macon Weekly Telegraph (Georgia)
New York Herald
New Orleans Tribune (Louisiana)
New Orleans Times (Louisiana)
Plaindealer (Detroit, MI)
Semi-Weekly Messenger (Wilmington, NC)
Washington Sentinel (DC)
Weekly Herald (New York)
Weekly Louisianian (New Orleans)

Manuscript and Archival Sources

Samuel Adolphus Cartwright 1793–1863 Family Papers. Mss. 2471, 2499, Louisiana and Lower Mississippi Valley Collections, LSU Libraries Special Collections, Hill Memorial Library, Louisiana State University, Baton Rouge.

Central Louisiana State Hospital Collections. Hill Memorial Library, Louisiana State University, Baton Rouge.

Joseph S. Copes Papers, 1831–1936. Collection 733, Louisiana Research Collection, Tulane University, New Orleans.

Eastern State Hospital Collection. Library of Virginia, Richmond.

French Society of New Orleans Collection. Hill Memorial Library, Louisiana State University, Baton Rouge.

Joseph Jones Papers. Mss. no. 468, Louisiana and Lower Mississippi Valley Collections, LSU Libraries Special Collections, Hill Memorial Library, Louisiana State University, Baton Rouge.

Kuntz Collection. Collection 600, Louisiana Research Collection, Tulane University, New Orleans.

Nell Battle Lewis Papers. North Carolina State Archives, Raleigh.

Office of the Governor Collections. North Carolina State Archives, Raleigh.

Benjamin Rush Papers, 1776–1812. Manuscript Division, MSS38547, Library of Congress, Washington, DC.

Western State Hospital Collection. Library of Virginia, Richmond.

Government Records

Abstract of the Returns of the Fifth Census, showing the Number of Free People, the Number of slaves, the federal or representative number and the aggregate of each county of each state of the United States. Prepared from the corrected returns of the Secretary of State to Congress, by the Clerk of the House of Representatives. Washington, DC: Duff Green, 1832.

De Bow, J. D. B. *Statistical view of the United States, embracing its territory, population— white, free colored, and slave—moral and social condition, industry, property and revenue; the detailed statistics of cities, towns, and counties; being a compendium of the seventh census; to which are added the results of every previous census, beginning with 1790,* Superintendent of the United States Census, Census Office. Washington, DC: Beverley Tucker, Senate Printer. 1854.

Dix, Dorothea. "Memorial to the Massachusetts Legislature (1843)." https://usa.usembassy.de/etexts/democrac/15.htm.

———. *Memorial of Miss D. L. Dix, to the Hon. the General Assembly in behalf of the insane of Maryland.* Maryland: General Assembly. House and Senate Documents, 1852.

———. *Memorial Soliciting Enlarged and Improved Accommodations for the Establishment of a New Hospital for the Insane of the State of Tennessee.* Nashville: General Assembly Press, 1847.

"Immigration and Insanity." In *Reports of the Immigration Commission,* vol. 2. Washington, DC: Government Printing Office, 1910.

John C. Calhoun to Richard Pakenham, Senate Documents, 28 Cong., 1st sess., 5053, April 18, 1844.

LOUISIANA

Annual Report of the Central Louisiana State Hospital, 1941 to the Governor. Baton Rouge: State Printing Press, 1941.

Report of the Board of Administrators of the Louisiana Hospital for Insane of the State of Louisiana, to the Governor, Biennial Period Ending March 31st, 1906. Baton Rouge: The Times, State Official Journal of Louisiana, 1906.

Report of the Board of Administrators of the Louisiana Hospital for Insane of the State of Louisiana, to the Governor, Biennial Period Ending March 31st, 1908. Baton Rouge: Daily State Publishing Co., 1908.

Report of the Board of Administrators of the Louisiana Hospital for Insane of the State of Louisiana, to the Governor, Biennial Period Ending March 31st, 1910. Baton Rouge: The New Advocate, Official Journal, 1910.

Report of the Board of Administrators of the Central Louisiana State Hospital of the State of Louisiana to the Governor, Biennial Period Ending March 31st, 1930. Alexandria: Standard Printing Co., 1930.

Report of the Board of the Administrators of the Central Louisiana State Hospital at Pineville, To his Excellency, the Governor, Biennial Period Ending March 31, 1934. Alexandria: Standard Printing Co., 1934.

NORTH CAROLINA

Annual Report of the Board of Directors and the Superintendent of the Eastern North Carolina Insane Asylum, for the Year ending December 31, 1882. Goldsboro, NC: Messenger Book and Job Printing House, 1883.

Report of the Eastern NC Insane Asylum for the Year of 1883. Goldsboro, NC: Messenger Steam Power Press Print, 1884.

Superintendent's Report of the Eastern NC Insane Asylum for the Year of 1884. Goldsboro, NC: Messenger Steam Power Press Print, 1885.

Superintendent's Report of the Eastern NC Insane Asylum, also the Reports of the Chairman of the Directors and of the State Treasurer, for the Year of 1886. Wilmington, NC: Messenger Steam Power Press Print, 1886. Reports for the years 1887, 1888, 1889 and 1890 were also consulted.

VIRGINIA

Annual Report of the Central Lunatic Asylum of the State of Virginia for the Fiscal Year Ending September 30, 1889. Richmond: J. H. O'Bannon, Superintendent of Public Printing, 1889. Reports for the following years were also consulted: 1891 and 1892.

Annual Report of the Central Lunatic Asylum of Virginia for the Fiscal Year 1886–1887. Richmond: A. R. Micou, Superintendent of Public Printing, 1887.

Annual Report of the Central State Hospital of the State of Virginia (Petersburg, VA.) for the Fiscal Year Ending September 30, 1895. Richmond: J. H. O'Bannon, Superintendent of Public Printing, 1895. Reports for the following years were also consulted: 1896 and 1898.

Fiftieth and Fifty-first Annual Reports of the Central State Hospital of Virginia (Petersburg) for the Fiscal Years Ending September 30, 1920 and 1921. Richmond: Davis Bottom, Superintendent of Public Printing, 1921.

Forty-Fifth Annual Report of the Central State Hospital of Virginia (Petersburg) for the Fiscal Year Ending September 30, 1915. Richmond: Davis Bottom, Superintendent of Public Printing, 1915.

Forty-Ninth Annual Report of the Central State Hospital of Virginia (Petersburg) for the Fiscal Year Ending September 30, 1919. Richmond: Davis Bottom, Superintendent of Public Printing, 1920.

The One Hundred and Forty-Sixth Annual Report of the Eastern State Hospital of Virginia (at Williamsburg) for the Fiscal Year Ending September 30, 1919. Richmond: Davis Bottom, Superintendent of Public Printing, 1919.

Report of the Board of Directors and Medical Superintendent of the Central Lunatic Asylum (for Colored Insane), Virginia, for the Year 1871–1872. Richmond: R. F. Walker, Superintendent of Public Printing, 1872. Reports for the years 1872–1873, 1877–1878, 1882–1883, and 1883–1884 were also consulted.

Thirty-First Annual Report of the Central State Hospital of Virginia (Petersburg) for the Fiscal Year Ending September 30, 1901. Richmond: J. H. O'Bannon: Superintendent of Public Printing, 1901.

Thirty-Fourth Annual Report of the Central State Hospital of Virginia (Petersburg) for the Fiscal Year Ending September 30, 1904 and Historical Sketch of Hospital. Richmond: J. H. O'Bannon: Superintendent of Public Printing, 1904.

Thirty-Sixth Annual Report of the Central State Hospital of Virginia (Petersburg) for the Fiscal Year Ending September 30, 1906. Richmond: Davis Bottom: Superintendent of Public Printing, 1906.

Published Primary Sources

Abraham, Karl. *Dreams and Myths: A Study in Race Psychology.* Trans. William A. White. New York: Journal of Nervous and Mental Disease Publishing, 1913.

"Académie royale des Sciences. Séance du 17 décembre. Population des États-Unis, Statistique médicale." *Archives générales de médecine* 30 (1832).

Adler, Alfred. *Über den nervosen Character.* Göttingen: Vandenhoeck & Ruprecht, 1912.

American Statistical Association. *Memorial of the American Statistical Association: Praying the Adoption of Measures for the Correction of Errors in the Returns of the Sixth Census.* Washington, DC: Gates and Seaton, 1844.

Andrews, Judson B. "The Distribution and Care of the Insane in the United States." *American Journal of Insanity* 44, no. 2 (1887): 192–211.

Bevis, William V. "Psychological Traits of the Southern Negro with Observations as to Some of His Psychoses." *American Journal of Psychiatry* 78 (1921–1922): 70–78.

"Black and White Insanity." *Charleston Mercury* (April 24, 1857): 1.

Blassingame, John W., ed. *Slave Testimony: Two Centuries of Letters, Speeches, Interviews, and Autobiographies*. Baton Rouge: Louisiana State University Press, 1977.

Caldwell, Charles. *Thoughts on the Original Unity of the Human Race*. Cincinnati: J. A. & U. P. James, 1852.

Calhoun, John C. "Speech on the Reception of Abolition Petitions." February 6, 1837. In *The Works of John C. Calhoun*, vol. 2, ed. Richard Kenner Crallé, 626–627. New York: D. Appleton, 1888.

———. "Ethnology of the Negro or Prognathous Race." *New Orleans Medical and Surgical Journal* 15 (January 1858): 149–163.

Cartwright, Samuel A. "Report on the Diseases and Physical Peculiarities of the Negro Race." *New Orleans Medical and Surgical Journal* 7 (May 1851): 691–715.

Chaillé, Stanford Emerson. "Intimidation and the Number of White and of Colored Voters in Louisiana in 1876." *New Orleans Medical and Surgical Journal* (1876).

———. *A Memoir of the Insane Asylum of the State of Louisiana, at Jackson*. Baton Rouge, LA: J. M. Taylor, 1858.

———. "Vital Statistics Applied to the Military-Reconstruction Politics of Louisiana." *New Orleans Medical and Surgical Journal* (1875).

"The Chamber of Commerce Declares Against Negro Domination." *Semi-Weekly Messenger* (Wilmington, NC), October 11, 1898.

Clarke, James Freeman. "Condition of the Free Colored People of the United States." *Christian Examiner* 29, no. 12 (March 25, 1859).

Deutsch, Albert. "The First U.S. Census of the Insane (1840) and Its Use as Pro-Slavery Propaganda." *Bulletin on the History of Medicine* 15 (January 1944): 469–482.

Diller, Theodore. "Causes of Insanity." *Pittsburgh Medical Review* 5 (October 1891): 295–296.

Drewry, William J. "Care and Condition of the Insane in Virginia." In *Proceedings of the National Conference of Charities and Correction*, ed. Alexander Johnson. Fort Wayne: Press of Fort Wayne Printing, 1908.

Du Bois, W. E. B. *The Gift of Black Folk: The Negroes in the Making of America*. Oxford: Oxford University Press, 2009.

Du Camp, Maxime. *Les Convulsions de Paris*. Paris: Librairie Hachette, 1878.

Dunbar, Paul Laurence. "Sympathy." *Lyrics of the Hearthside*. New York: Dodd, Mead & Co., 1899.

Dunglison, Robley. "Dr. Dunglinson's Statistics of Insanity in the United States." *American Journal of Insanity* (1860).

Evarts, Arrah B. "Dementia Praecox in the Colored Race." *Psychoanalytic Review* 1, no. 4 (October 1914).

———. "The Ontogenetic Against the Phylogenetic Elements in the Psychoses of the Colored Race." *Psychoanalytic Review* 3 (1916).

"Facts Worth Noticing." *Macon Weekly Telegraph* (November 4, 1856): 3

"Freedom and the Negro." *The Conservative* (June 14, 1900): 4.

Green, E. M. "Manic-Depressive Psychosis in the Negro." *American Journal of Insanity* 73 (1917): 619–626.

———. "Psychoses Among Negroes—A Comparative Study." *Journal of Nervous and Mental Disease* 41, no. 11 (1914): 697–708.

Grier, S. L. "The Negro and His Diseases." *New Orleans Medical and Surgical Journal* 9 (January 1853): 752–763.

Havelock Ellis, Henry. "Sexual Inversion in Women." *Alienist and Neurologist* 16 (1895): 143–144.

Hodges, J. Addison. "The Effect of Freedom upon the Physical and Psychological Development of the Negro." *Virginia Medical Semi-Monthly* 5 (May 1900): 106–110.

Holcombe, William H. "The Alternative: A Separate Nationality or the Africanization of the South." *Southern Literary Messenger* 32, no. 2 (February 1861): 81–88.

Hughes, Langston. "Black Workers." Excerpts. *The Crisis: A Record of the Darker Races* 40, no. 4 (April 1933).

Hurmence, Belinda, ed. *Before Freedom, When I Just Can Remember: Twenty-Seven Oral Histories of Former South Carolina Slaves.* Winston-Salem, NC: John F. Blair, 2000.

Jarvis, Edward. "Statistics of Insanity in the United States." *Boston Medical and Surgical Journal* 27 (September 21, 1842): 116–121.

Jefferson, Thomas. *Notes on the State of Virginia.* London: John Stockdale, 1787.

Jones, Joseph. *General Medicine, Diseases of the Nervous System by Joseph Jones, M.D., Delivered Before the Louisiana State Medical Society at its 11th Annual Session, New Orleans, LA, April 1889.* New Orleans: L. Graham and Son, 1889.

Jung, Carl. "Letter from Doctor Jung." *Psychoanalytic Review* 1, no. 1 (November 1913): 117–118.

King, Martin Luther, Jr. "MLK at Western." December 18, 1963. Western Michigan University Archives and Regional History Collections and University Libraries, Western Michigan University. http://wmich.edu/sites/default/files/attachments/MLK.pdf.

Lind, John E. "The Color Complex in the Negro." *Psychoanalytic Review* 1, no. 4 (October 1914).

———. "Diagnostic Pitfalls in the Examinations of Negroes." *New York Medical Journal* 99, no. 26 (1914): 1286–1287.

———. "The Dream as a Simple Wish-Fulfillment in the Negro." *Psychoanalytic Review* 1, no. 3 (1913).

Meigs, Charles D. "Article XII: Extract from a Memoir of Samuel George Morton, M.D., Late President of the Academy of Natural Sciences of Philadelphia." *American Journal of Science* 13, no. 38 (May 1852): 153–178.

Miller, John Fulenwider. "The Effects of Emancipation upon the Mental and Physical Health of the Negro of the South." *North Carolina Medical Journal* 38 (December 1896): 287–294.

Monette, John W. *An Essay on Causes of the Variety of Complexion and Form of the Human Species*, 1824, Mss. 593, Louisiana and Lower Mississippi Valley Collections, LSU Libraries Special Collections, Louisiana State University Libraries, Baton Rouge.

Morton, Samuel George. *Crania Ægyptiaca: Observations on Egyptian Ethnography, Derived from Anatomy, History and the Monuments*. Philadelphia: John Pennington, 1844.

———. *Crania Americana: or, a Comparative View of the Skulls of Various Aboriginal Nations of North and South America*. Philadelphia: J. Dobson, 1839.

———. *An Inquiry into the Distinctive Characteristics of the Aboriginal Race of America*. Philadelphia: John Pennington, 1844.

Olmsted, Frederick Law. *A Journey in the Back Country*. New York: Mason Brothers, 1860.

O'Malley, Mary. "Psychoses in the Colored Race: A Study in Comparative Psychiatry." *American Journal of Insanity* 71 (1914): 309–337.

Overton, William M., Charles Maurice Smith, and Beverley Tucker. "Slaves and Free Negroes." *Washington Sentinel*, September 1, 1854.

Pinel, Philippe. *Traité médico-philosophique sur l'aliénation mentale, Seconde édition, entièrement refondue et très-augmentée*. Paris: J. Ant. Brosson, 1809.

Prudhomme, Charles. "The Problem of Suicide in the American Negro." *Psychoanalytic Review* 25 (1938): 187–204.

"Reflections on the Census of 1840." *Southern Literary Messenger* 9 (June 1843): 340–352.

Rush, Benjamin. *Medical Inquiries and Observations upon the Diseases of the Mind*. Philadelphia: Kimber & Richardson, 1812.

Sagra, Ramón de la. "Statistique des aliénés et des sourds-muets dans les États-Unis de l'Amérique du Nord." *Annales Médico-Psychologiques* 1 (1843): 281–283.

"The Sixth Census of the United States." *Hunt's Merchants' Magazine* 12 (1845).

Smith, James McCune "Freedom and Slavery for Afric-Americans (1844)." In *The Works of James McCune Smith: Black Intellectual and Abolitionist*, ed. John Stauffer, 61–65. Oxford: Oxford University Press, 2006.

Smith, Samuel Stanhope. *Essay on the Causes of Variety of Complexion and Figure in the Human Species*. New Brunswick: L. Simpson & Co., 1810.

"Southern Medical Reports." *De Bow's Review* 9, no. 3 (September 1850).

"State Board of Charities Calls Upon the People to Help the Insane." *The Caucasian* 15, no. 2 (March 29, 1900).

"Statistics of Affliction." *Weekly Louisianian* (November 30, 1871): 4.

Thompson, James Lawrence. *Shattered Minds: Fifty Years at the South Carolina State Hospital for the Insane.* Columbia: South Carolina Department of Mental Health, 1989.

Tiffany, Francis. *Life of Dorothea Lynde Dix.* Boston: Houghton, Mifflin, 1890.

"Unity of the Human Race Disproved by the Hebrew Bible." *De Bow's Review* 4, no. 2 (August 1860): 129–136.

Waldo, J. Curtis. *Illustrated Visitor's Guide to New Orleans.* New Orleans, LA: J. Curtis Waldo, 1879.

White, William Alanson. *Mental Mechanisms.* New York: Journal of Nervous and Mental Disease Publishing, 1911.

———. *Outlines of Psychiatry.* New York: Journal of Nervous and Mental Disease Publishing, 1911.

———. *Thoughts of a Psychiatrist on the War and After.* New York: P. B. Hoeber, 1919.

Witmer, A. H. "Insanity in the Colored Race in the United States." *Alienist and Neurologist* 12 (1891): 19–30.

Woodruff, L. "The Seventh United States Census." *Hunt's Merchants' Magazine* 34 (February 1856): 171–173.

Secondary Sources

Abbott, Andrew. *The System of Professions: An Essay on the Division of Expert Labor.* Chicago: University of Chicago Press, 1988.

Alston, Lee J., and Joseph P. Ferrie. *Southern Paternalism and the American Welfare State: Economics, Politics, and Institutions in the South, 1865–1965.* Cambridge: Cambridge University Press, 1999.

Anderson, James. *The Education of Blacks in the South, 1860–1935.* Chapel Hill: University of North Carolina Press, 2010.

Anderson, Margo, and Stephen E. Fienberg. *Who Counts? The Politics of Census-Taking in Contemporary America.* New York: Russell Sage Foundation, 2001.

Araujo, Ana Lucia. *Museums and Atlantic Slavery.* New York: Routledge, 2020.

———. *Slavery in the Age of Memory: Engaging the Past.* New York: Bloomsbury, 2020.

Ash, Mitchell G. "Americanizing Psychoanalysis." *Modern Intellectual History* 14, no. 2 (August 2017): 607–617.

Ash, Stephen V. *A Massacre in Memphis: The Race Riot That Shook the Nation One Year After the Civil War.* New York: Hill and Wang, 2014.

———. *When the Yankees Came: Conflict and Chaos in the Occupied South, 1861–1865.* Chapel Hill: University of North Carolina Press, 1995.

Ayers, Edward L. *The Promise of the New South: Life After Reconstruction.* Oxford: Oxford University Press, 1992.

Baker, Lee D. *From Savage to Negro: Anthropology and the Construction of Race, 1896–1954.* Berkeley: University of California Press, 1998.

Baker, Robert B., Harriet A. Washington, Ololade Olakanmi, Todd L. Savitt, Elizabeth A. Jacobs, Eddie Hoover, and Matthew K. Wynia. "African American Physicians and Organized Medicine, 1846–1968: Origins of a Racial Divide." *Journal of the American Medical Association* 300, no. 3 (2008): 306–313.

Baldwin, James. *I Am Not Your Negro: A Major Motion Picture Directed by Raoul Peck.* New York: Vintage Books, 2017.

Bankole-Medina, Katherine. *Slavery and Medicine: Enslavement and Medical Practices in Antebellum Louisiana.* New York: Taylor and Francis, 1998.

Baptist, Edward. *The Half Has Never Been Told: Slavery and the Making of American Capitalism.* London: Hachette, 2016.

Barreyre, Nicolas. "Réunifier l'Union: intégrer l'Ouest à la Reconstruction américaine, 1870–1872." *Revue d'Histoire Moderne et Contemporaine* 49, no. 4 (Autumn 2002): 7–36.

Bean, Christopher B. *Too Great a Burden to Bear: The Struggle and Failure of the Freedmen's Bureau in Texas.* New York: Fordham University Press, 2016.

Beckert, Sven. *Empire of Cotton: A Global History.* New York: Knopf Doubleday, 2014.

Beckert, Sven, and Seth Rickman, eds. *Slavery's Capitalism: A New History of American Economic Development.* Philadelphia: University of Pennsylvania Press, 2016.

Berlin, Ira. *Generations of Captivity: A History of African-American Slaves.* Cambridge, MA: Belknap Press of Harvard University Press, 2003.

Berry, Daina Ramey. *The Price for Their Pound of Flesh: The Value of the Enslaved, from Womb to Grave, in the Building of a Nation.* Boston: Beacon Press, 2017.

Bischoff Paulus, Sarah. "America's Long Eulogy for Compromise: Henry Clay and American Politics, 1854–58." *Journal of the Civil War Era* 4, no. 1 (2014): 28–52.

Blackett, Richard J. "Dispossessing Massa: Fugitive Slaves and the Politics of Slavery After 1850." *American Nineteenth Century History* 10, no. 2 (2009): 119–136.

Blackmon, Douglas A. *Slavery by Another Name: The Re-enslavement of Black Americans from the Civil War to World War II.* New York: Anchor, 2009.

Blakey, Robert, and Judith Harrington. *Bones in the Basement: Postmodern Racism in Nineteenth-Century Medical Training.* Washington, DC: Smithsonian Institution Press, 1997.

Blassingame, John W. *Black New Orleans, 1860–1880.* Chicago: University of Chicago Press, 1973.

Boster, Dea H. *African American Slavery and Disability: Bodies, Property, and Power in the Antebellum South, 1800–1860.* New York: Routledge, 2014.

Branam, Chris W. "'The Africans Have Taken Arkansas': Political Activities of African Americans in the Reconstruction Legislature." *Arkansas Historical Quarterly* 73, no. 3 (Autumn 2014): 233–267.

Branson, Susan. "Phrenology and the Science of Race in Antebellum America." *Early American Studies* 15, no. 1 (2017): 164–193.

Brophy, Alfred. *University, Court, and Slave: Pro-slavery Thought in Southern Colleges and Courts and the Coming of Civil War.* Oxford: Oxford University Press, 2016.

Browne, Hugh M. "Method of Education and Teaching for the Children of Undeveloped Races." *Southern Workman and Hampton School Record: 1899.* Hampton, VA: Hampton Normal and Agricultural Institute, 1899.

Brundage, W. Fitzhugh. *Lynching in the New South: Georgia and Virginia, 1880–1930.* Urbana: University of Illinois Press, 1993.

Bryan, Charles S. *Asylum Doctor: James Woods Babcock and the Red Plague of Pellagra.* Columbia: University of South Carolina Press, 2014.

Burawoy, Michael. "For Public Sociology." *American Sociological Review* 70, no. 1 (February 2005): 4–28.

Burg, Robert W. "Amnesty, Civil Rights, and the Meaning of Liberal Republicanism, 1862–1872." *American Nineteenth Century History* 4, no. 3 (Fall 2003): 29–60.

Campbell Bartoletti, Susan. *Black Potatoes: The Story of the Great Irish Famine, 1845–1850.* Boston: Houghton Mifflin Harcourt, 2014.

Caplan, Ruth B. *Psychiatry and the Community in Nineteenth-Century America: The Recurring Concern with the Environment in the Prevention and Treatment of Mental Illness.* New York: Basic Books, 1969.

Carden, Art, and Christopher J. Coyne. "The Political Economy of the Reconstruction Era's Race Riots." *Public Choice* 157, no. 1–2 (October 2013): 57–71.

Carlson, Leonard A., and Mark A. Roberts. "Indian Lands, 'Squatterism,' and Slavery: Economic Interests and the Passage of the Indian Removal Act of 1830." *Explorations in Economic History* 43, no. 3 (2006): 486–504.

Carpenter-Song, Elizabeth A., Meghan Nordquest Schwallie, and Jeffrey Longhoffer. "Cultural Competence Reexamined: Critique and Directions for the Future." *Psychiatric Services* 58, no. 10 (October 2007): 1362–1365.

Cassanello, Robert. *To Render Invisible: Jim Crow and Public Life in New South Jacksonville.* Gainesville: University of Florida Press, 2013.

Cassedy, J. H. "Medical World of Madness, Morality, and Number." *Reviews in American History* 7 (June 1979): 219–223.

Castel, Robert. *L'Ordre psychiatrique.* Paris: Éditions de Minuit, 1976.

Castles, Katherine. "Quiet Eugenics: Sterilization in North Carolina's Institutions for the Mentally Retarded, 1945–1965." *Journal of Southern History* 68, no. 4 (November 2002): 849–878.

Cecelski, David. *Along Freedom Road: Hyde County, North Carolina, and the Fate of Black Schools in the South*. Chapel Hill: University of North Carolina Press, 1994.

Childers, Christopher. *The Failure of Popular Sovereignty: Slavery, Manifest Destiny, and the Radicalization of Southern Politics*. Lawrence: University Press of Kansas, 2012.

Chodoff, Paul. "Hysteria and Women." *American Journal of Psychiatry* 139, no. 5 (1982): 545–551.

Claeys, Gregory. "The 'Survival of the Fittest' and the Origins of Social Darwinism." *Journal of the History of Ideas* 61, no. 2 (April 2000): 223–240.

Clarke, Erskine. *Dwelling Place: A Plantation Epic*. New Haven, CT: Yale University Press, 2005.

Cloyd, Benjamin G. *Haunted by Atrocity: Civil War Prisons in American Memory*. Baton Rouge: Louisiana State University Press, 2010.

Clymer Bigelow, Ann. "Insanity in Civil War Ohio." *Ohio Valley History* 17, no. 2 (2017): 46–64.

Cobb, Michael D., and Jeffery A. Jenkins. "Race and the Representation of Blacks' Interests During Reconstruction." *Political Research Quarterly* 54, no. 1 (March 2001): 181–204.

Cohen, Patricia Cline. *A Calculating People: The Spread of Numeracy in Early America*. Chicago: University of Chicago Press, 1988.

Colucci, Mario. "Hystériques, internés, hommes infâmes: Michel Foucault et la résistance au pouvoir." *Sud/Nord* 1, no. 20 (2005): 123–145.

Cooper, Anastasia. "The Ongoing Correctional Chaos in Criminalizing Mental Illness: The Realignment's Effects on California Jails." *Hastings Women's Law Journal* 24, no. 2 (2013): 339–361.

Cooper, Brittney. *Eloquent Rage: A Black Feminist Discovers Her Superpower*. New York: St. Martin's Press, 2018.

Cooper Owens, Deirdre. *Medical Bondage: Race, Gender, and the Origins of American Gynecology*. Athens: University of Georgia Press, 2016.

Correia, David. "Making Destiny Manifest: United States Territorial Expansion and the Dispossession of Two Mexican Property Claims in New Mexico, 1824–1899." *Journal of Historical Geography* 35, no. 1 (January 2009): 87–103.

Couturier, Lydie. "L'enfermement des aliénés: l'asile de Stephansfeld (Bas-Rhin, 1835–1860) et la loi de 1838." *Revue d'Histoire de la Protection Sociale* 7, no. 1 (January 2014): 58–79.

Crespino, Joseph. *In Search of Another Country: Mississippi and the Conservative Counterrevolution*. Princeton, NJ: Princeton University Press, 2007.

Cresswell, Stephen. *Rednecks, Redeemers, and Race: Mississippi after Reconstruction, 1877–1917*. Jackson: University Press of Mississippi, 2006.

Cruz, Barbara C., Michael J. Berson, and Donald Falls. "Swimming Not Allowed:

Teaching About Segregated Public Beaches and Pools." *Social Studies* 103, no. 6 (November–December 2012): 252–259.

Dain, Norman. *Concepts of Insanity in the United States, 1789–1865.* New Brunswick, NJ: Rutgers University Press, 1964.

———. *Disordered Minds: The First Century of Eastern State Hospital in Williamsburg, Virginia, 1766–1866.* Charlottesville: University Press of Virginia, 1971.

Davis, Angela Y. *Women, Race & Class.* New York: Vintage, 1983.

Davis, James F. *Who Is Black? One Nation's Definition.* University Park: Pennsylvania State University Press, 2001.

DeLatte, Carolyn E. "The St. Landry Riot: A Forgotten Incident of Reconstruction Violence." *Louisiana History: The Journal of the Louisiana Historical Association* 17, no. 1 (Winter 1976): 41–49.

DeVries, Marten W., Norbert Müller, Hans-Jürgen Möller, and Lettew F. Saugstad. "Emil Kraepelin's Legacy: Systematic Clinical Observation and the Categorical Classification of Psychiatric Diseases." *European Archives of Psychiatry and Clinical Neuroscience* 258, suppl. 2 (2008): 1–2.

Deyle, Steve. *Carry Me Back: The Domestic Slave Trade in American Life.* New York: Oxford University Press, 2005.

Di Vittorio, Pierangelo. "De la psychiatrie à la biopolitique, ou la naissance de l'État bio-sécuritaire." In *Michel Foucault et le contrôle social,* ed. Alain Beaulieu, 911–924. Laval: Presses de l'Université de Laval, 2005.

Donohue, John J., III, James J. Heckman, and Petra E. Todd. "The Schooling of Southern Blacks: The Roles of Legal Activism and Private Philanthropy, 1910–1960." *Quarterly Journal of Economics* 117, no. 1 (February 2002): 225–268.

Doolen, Andy. *Fugitive Empire: Locating Early American Imperialism.* Minneapolis: University of Minnesota Press, 2005.

Dorlin, Elsa. *La matrice de la race: Généalogie sexuelle et coloniale de la nation française.* Paris: La Découverte, 2008.

Dorr, Gregory Michael. *Segregation's Science: Eugenics and Society in Virginia.* Charlottesville: University of Virginia Press, 2008.

Downs, Jim. *Maladies of Empire: How Colonialism, Slavery, and War Transformed Medicine.* Cambridge, MA: Harvard University Press, 2021.

———. *Sick from Freedom: African American Illness and Suffering During the Civil War and Reconstruction.* Oxford: Oxford University Press, 2015.

Doyle, Dennis. *Psychiatry and Racial Liberalism in Harlem, 1936–1968.* Rochester, NY: University of Rochester Press, 2016.

Driggers, Edward Allen. "The Chemistry of Blackness: Benjamin Rush, Thomas Jefferson, Everard Home, and the Project of Defining Blackness Through Chemical Explanations." *Critical Philosophy of Race* 7, no. 2 (July 2019): 372–391.

Du Bois, W. E. B. *Black Reconstruction in America: An Essay Toward a History of the Part Which Black Folk Played in the Attempt to Reconstruct Democracy in America, 1860– 1880.* New York: Harcourt, Brace, 1935.

Duffy, John. *The Rudolph Matas History of Medicine in Louisiana.* Gretna: Pelican, 1976.

Dwyer, Ellen. "A Historical Perspective." In *Sex Roles and Psychopathology,* ed. Cathy Widom, 19–48. Berlin: Springer, 2013.

Earle, Jonathan, and Diane Mutti Burke, eds. *Bleeding Kansas, Bleeding Missouri: The Long Civil War on the Border.* Topeka: University of Kansas Press, 2013.

Edwards, Laura. "Captives of Wilmington: The Riot and Historical Memories of Political Conflict, 1865–1898." In *Democracy Betrayed: The Wilmington Race Riot of 1898 and Its Legacy,* ed. David S. Cecelski and Timothy B. Tyson, 107–130. Chapel Hill: University of North Carolina Press, 2000.

Edwards-Grossi, Élodie. *Bad Brains: La psychiatrie et la lutte des Noirs américains pour la justice raciale, XXe–XXIe siècles.* Rennes: Presses universitaires de Rennes, 2021.

Equal Justice Initiative. *Lynching in America: Confronting the Legacy of Racial Terror.* 3rd ed. Montgomery, AL: Equal Justice Initiative, 2017. https://lynchinginamerica.eji .org/report.

Etcheson, Nicole. "'Our lives, our fortunes and our sacred honors': The Kansas Civil War and the Revolutionary." *American Nineteenth Century History* 1, no. 1 (Spring 2000): 62–81.

Eyal, Gil. "For a Sociology of Expertise: The Social Origins of the Autism Epidemic." *American Journal of Sociology* 118, no. 4 (January 2013): 863–907.

Fett, Sharla. *Working Cures: Healing, Health, and Power on Southern Slave Plantations.* Chapel Hill: University of North Carolina Press, 2002.

Finnegan, Terence. "Lynching and Political Power in Mississippi and South Carolina." In *Under Sentence of Death: Lynching in the South,* ed. W. Fitzhugh Brundage, 189– 218. Chapel Hill: University of North Carolina Press, 1997.

Foner, Eric. "The Wilmot Proviso Revisited." *Journal of American History* 56, no. 2 (September 1969): 262–279.

Foucault, Michel. *Histoire de la Folie à l'Âge Classique.* Paris: Gallimard, 1972.

——— *Il faut défendre la société: Cours au Collège de France, 1975–1976.* Paris: Le Seuil, 1997.

———. *Le Pouvoir psychiatrique: Cours au Collège de France, 1973–1974.* Paris: Le Seuil, 2003.

Fox-Amato, Matthew. *Exposing Slavery: Photography, Human Bondage, and the Birth of Modern Visual Politics in America.* Oxford: Oxford University Press, 2019.

Fredrickson, George M. *The Black Image in the White Mind: The Debate on Afro- American Character and Destiny, 1817–1914.* New York: Harper & Row, 1971.

Freidson, Eliot. *Profession of Medicine: A Study of the Sociology of Applied Knowledge.* Chicago: University of Chicago Press, 1970.

Gambino, Matthew. "Fevered Decisions: Race, Ethics, and Clinical Vulnerability in the Malarial Treatment of Neurosyphilis, 1922–1953." *Hastings Center Report* 45, no. 4 (July–August 2015): 39–50.

———. "'The Savage Heart Beneath the Civilized Exterior': Race, Citizenship, and Mental Illness in Washington, DC, 1900–1940." *Disability Studies Quarterly* 28, no. 3 (Summer 2008).

———. "'These strangers within our gates': Race, Psychiatry and Mental Illness Among Black Americans at St. Elizabeths Hospital in Washington, DC, 1900–40." *History of Psychiatry* 19, no. 4 (December 2008): 387–408.

Gamble, Vanessa N. *Making A Place for Ourselves: The Black Hospital Movement, 1920–1945.* New York: Oxford University Press, 1995.

Garland, Joseph. "The Boston Medical and Surgical Journal, 1828–1928." *New England Journal of Medicine* 198, no. 1 (January 1928): 1–13.

Genovese, Eugene. *Roll, Jordan, Roll: The World the Slaves Made.* New York: Vintage, 1976.

Gilman, Sander L. *Difference and Pathology: Stereotypes of Sexuality, Race, and Madness.* Ithaca, NY: Cornell University Press, 1985.

———. *Freud, Race, and Gender.* Princeton, NJ: Princeton University Press, 1995.

Gilmore, Glenda. *Gender and Jim Crow: Women and the Politics of White Supremacy in North Carolina, 1896–1920.* Chapel Hill: University of North Carolina Press, 1996.

Glymph, Thavolia. "The Second Middle Passage: The Transition from Slavery to Freedom at Davis Bend, Mississippi." PhD diss., Purdue University, 1994.

Goffman, Erving. *Asylums: Essays on the Social Situation of Mental Patients and Other Inmates.* Chicago: Aldine Transaction, 1968.

———. *The Presentation of Self in Everyday Life.* Edinburgh: University of Edinburg Social Sciences Research Centre, 1956.

Gonaver, Wendy. *The Peculiar Institution and the Making of Modern Psychiatry, 1840–1880.* Chapel Hill: University of North Carolina Press, 2019.

Gordon, Linda. *The Second Coming of the KKK: The Ku Klux Klan of the 1920s and the American Political Tradition.* New York: Liveright, 2017.

Greene, Talya. "The Kraepelinian Dichotomy: The Twin Pillars Crumbling?" *History of Psychiatry* 18, no. 3 (2007): 361–379.

Grob, Gerald. "Edward Jarvis and the Federal Census." *Bulletin of the History of Medicine* 50 (Spring 1976): 4–27.

———. *Edward Jarvis and the Medical World of Nineteenth-Century America.* Knoxville: University of Tennessee Press, 1978.

———. *The Inner World of American Psychiatry, 1890–1940.* New Brunswick, NJ: Rutgers University Press, 1985.

————. *Mad Among Us*. New York: Simon and Schuster, 1994.

————. *Mental Illness and American Society, 1875–1940*. Princeton, NJ: Princeton University Press, 1987.

————. *Mental Institutions in America: Social Policy to 1875*. New York: Free Press, 1973.

Grossi, Élodie. "Behind the Hospitals' Closed Doors: Medical Archives as Sites of Racial Memory and Social (In)Justice." *Revue Française d'Études Américaines* 162, no. 1 (January 2020): 35–50.

————. "Médicaliser la folle Émancipation, soigner la folie noire? Le contexte d'ouverture du Central Lunatic State Asylum for Colored Insane en question." In *Imaginaire racial et oppositions identitaires (aire anglophone)*, ed. Michel Prum, 237–249. Paris: L'Harmattan, 2016.

————. "Truth in Numbers? Emancipation, Race, and Federal Census Statistics in the Debates over Black Mental Health in the United States, 1840–1900." *Endeavour* 45, no. 1–2 (March 2021): 1–10.

Grossman, James. *Land of Hope: Chicago, Black Southerners, and the Great Migration*. Chicago: University of Chicago Press, 1989.

Grossman, Pam. "Responding to Our Critics: From Crisis to Opportunity in Research on Teacher Education." *Journal of Teacher Education* 59, no. 1 (January 2008): 10–23.

Hale, Grace Elizabeth. *Making Whiteness: The Culture of Segregation in the South, 1890–1940*. New York: Pantheon, 1998.

Haller, John S., Jr. "The Negro and the Southern Physician: A Study of Medical and Racial Attitudes, 1800–1860." *Medical History* 16 (July 1972): 238–253.

Hansen, Helena, Philippe Bourgois, and Ernest Drucker. "Pathologizing Poverty: New Forms of Diagnosis, Disability, and Structural Stigma Under Welfare Reform." *Social Science & Medicine* 103 (February 2014): 76–83.

Hardwick, Kevin R. "'Your Old Father Abe Lincoln Is Dead and Damned': Black Soldiers and the Memphis Race Riot of 1866." *Journal of Social History* 27, no. 1 (Autumn 1993): 109–128.

Harris, James. "Pinel Orders the Chains Removed from the Insane at Bicêtre." *Archives of General Psychiatry* 60, no. 5 (2003): 442–456.

Harris, Trudier. *Exorcising Blackness: Historical and Literary Lynching and Burning Rituals*. Bloomington: Indiana University Press, 1984.

Haynes, Stephen R. *Noah's Curse: The Biblical Justification of American Slavery*. Oxford: Oxford University Press, 2002.

Healy, David. *The Antidepressant Era*. Cambridge, MA: Harvard University Press, 1997.

Highsmith, Andrew R., and Ansley T. Erickson. "Segregation as Splitting, Segregation as Joining: Schools, Housing, and the Many Modes of Jim Crow." *American Journal of Education* 121, no. 4 (August 2015): 563–595.

Hirsch, Arnold. *Making the Second Ghetto*. Chicago: University of Chicago Press, 1998.

Hirshbein, Laura D. "Science, Gender, and the Emergence of Depression in American Psychiatry, 1952–1980." *Journal of the History of Medicine and Allied Sciences* 61, no. 2 (2006): 196–216.

Hobbs, Allyson. *A Chosen Exile: A History of Racial Passing in American Life*. Cambridge, MA: Harvard University Press, 2014.

Hoberman, John. *Black and Blue: The Origins and Consequences of Medical Racism*. Berkeley: University of California Press, 2012.

Hodes, Martha. *White Women, Black Men: Illicit Sex in the Nineteenth-Century South*. New Haven, CT: Yale University Press, 1997.

Hoff, Paul. "The Kraepelinian Tradition." *Dialogues in Clinical Neuroscience* 17, no. 1 (2005): 31–41.

Hofstadter, Richard. "From Calhoun to the Dixiecrats." *Social Research* 82, no. 1 (Spring 2015): 245–261.

Hogarth, Rana. *Medicalizing Blackness: Making Racial Difference in the Atlantic World, 1780–1840*. Chapel Hill: University of North Carolina Press, 2017.

Hollis, Shirley A. "Neither Slave nor Free: The Ideology of Capitalism and the Failure of Radical Reform in the American South." *Critical Sociology* 35, no. 1 (2009): 9–27.

Holloway, Pippa. *Sexuality, Politics, and Social Control in Virginia, 1920–1945*. Chapel Hill: University of North Carolina Press, 2006.

Hudson, Nicholas. "From 'Nation' to 'Race': The Origin of Racial Classification in Eighteenth-Century Thought." *Eighteenth-Century Studies* 29, no. 3 (Spring 1996): 247–264.

Humphreys, Margaret. *Intensely Human: The Health of the Black Soldier in the American Civil War*. Baltimore: Johns Hopkins University Press, 2008.

Huret, Romain. *American Tax Resisters*. Cambridge, MA: Harvard University Press, 2014.

———. *La fin de la pauvreté? Les experts sociaux et la Guerre contre la pauvreté aux États-Unis (1945–1974)*. Paris: EHESS, 2008.

Jackson, Luther P. *Negro Office-Holders in Virginia, 1865–1895*. Norfolk, VA: Guide Quality Press, 1945.

Jeliffe, Smith Ely, and William Alanson White. *Diseases of the Nervous System: A Text-Book of Neurology and Psychiatry*. Philadelphia: Lea and Febinger, 1915.

Jennings, Thelma. "'Us Colored Women Had to Go Though a Plenty': Sexual Exploitation of African-American Slave Women." *Journal of Women's History* 1, no. 3 (1990): 45–74.

Joinson, Carla. *Vanished in Hiawatha: The Story of the Canton Asylum for Insane Indians*. Lincoln: University of Nebraska Press, 2016.

Johnson, Walter. *River of Dark Dreams: Slavery and Empire in the Cotton Kingdom*. Cambridge, MA: Harvard University Press, 2013.

Jones, Marian Moser. "Creating a Science of Homelessness During the Reagan Era." *Milbank Quarterly* 93, no. 1 (March 2015): 139–178.

Jones, William P. *The March on Washington: Jobs, Freedom, and the Forgotten History of Civil Rights.* New York: W. W. Norton, 2013.

Jones-Rogers, Stephanie. "'She could . . . spare one ample breast for the profit of her owner': White Mothers and Enslaved Wet Nurses' Invisible Labor in American Slave Markets." *Slavery & Abolition* 38, no. 2 (2017): 1–19.

Jordan, Winthrop D. "Historical Origins of the One-Drop Racial Rule in the United States." *Journal of Critical Mixed Race Studies* 1, no. 1 (2014): 98–132.

———. *White over Black: American Attitudes Toward the Negro, 1550–1812.* Chapel Hill: University of North Carolina Press, 2013.

Kaneko, Ayumu. "The Politics of the Black Rapist Myth: American Racial Violence, Gender and Class at the Turn of the 20th Century." *J-Stage* 3 (2007): 5–18.

Kantrowitz, Stephen. *Ben Tillman and the Reconstruction of White Supremacy.* Chapel Hill: University of North Carolina Press, 2000.

Katz, Michael B. *Poverty and Policy in American History.* New York: Academic Press, 1983.

Keel, Terence D. "Religion, Polygenism and the Early Science of Human Origins." *History of the Human Sciences* 26, no. 2 (April 2013): 3–32.

Keele, Luke, William Cubbison, and Ismail White. "Suppressing Black Votes: A Historical Case Study of Voting Restrictions in Louisiana." *American Political Science Review* 115, no. 2 (March 2021): 694–700.

Keith, LeeAnna. *The Colfax Massacre: The Untold Story of Black Power, White Terror, and the Death of Reconstruction.* New York: Oxford University Press, 2008.

Kennedy, Angie C. "Eugenics, 'Degenerate Girls,' and Social Workers During the Progressive Era." *Affilia* 23, no. 1 (February 2008): 22–37.

Kenny, Stephen C. "The Development of Medical Museums in the Antebellum American South: Slave Bodies in Networks of Anatomical Exchange." *Bulletin of the History of Medicine* 87, no. 1 (Spring 2013): 32–62.

———. "'A Dictate of Both Interest and Mercy'? Slave Hospitals in the Antebellum South." *Journal of the History of Medicine and Allied Sciences* 65, no. 1 (January 2010): 2–47.

———. "Medical Racism's Poison Pen: The Toxic World of Dr. Henry Ramsay (1821–1856)." *Southern Quarterly* 53 (Spring–Summer 2016): 70–96.

———. "Power, Opportunism, Racism: Human Experiments Under American Slavery." *Endeavour* 39, no. 1 (2015): 10–20.

King, Marissa D., and Heather A. Haveman. "Antislavery in America: The Press, the Pulpit, and the Rise of Antislavery Societies." *Administrative Science Quarterly* 53, no. 3 (September 2008): 492–528.

Kirby, Jack T. "Black and White in the Rural South, 1915–1954." *Agricultural History* 58, no. 3 (July 1984): 411–422.

Kirmayer, Laurence J. "Rethinking Cultural Competence." *Transcultural Psychiatry* 49, no. 2 (2012): 149–164.

Koger, Larry. *Black Slaveowners: Free Black Slave Masters in South Carolina, 1790–1860.* Jefferson, NC: McFarland, 2010.

Kraam, Abdullah. "Karl Ludwig Kahlbaum by Dr. Ewald Hecker (1899)." *History of Psychiatry* 19, no. 1 (2008): 77–80.

Krieger, Nancy. "Shades of Difference: Theoretical Underpinnings of the Medical Controversy on Black/White Differences in the United States 1830–1870." *International Journal of Health Services* 17, no. 2 (January 1987): 259–278.

Lande, R. Gregory. *Madness, Malingering, and Malfeasance: The Transformation of Psychiatry and the Law in the Civil War Era.* Lincoln, NE: Potomac Books, 2005.

Landers, Jane G., ed. *Against the Odds: Free Blacks in the Slave Societies of the Americas.* New York: Routledge, 2013.

Lawson, William B., Nancy Hepler, and Jack Holladay. "Race as a Factor in Inpatient and Outpatient Admissions and Diagnosis." *Psychiatric Services* 45, no. 1 (April 1994): 72–74.

LeFlouria, Talitha L. *Chained in Silence: Black Women and Convict Labor in the New South.* Chapel Hill: University of North Carolina Press, 2015.

Lewis, Glyn, Caroline Croft-Jeffreys, and Anthony David. "Are British Psychiatrists Racist?" *British Journal of Psychiatry* 157, no. 3 (September 1990): 410–415.

Lichtenstein, Alex. *Twice the Work of Free Labor: The Political Economy of Convict Labor in the New South.* London: Verso, 1996.

Lindquist, Wendi A. "Stealing from the Dead: Scientists, Settlers, and Indian Burial Sites in Early-Nineteenth-Century Oregon." *Oregon Historical Quarterly* 115, no. 3 (Fall 2014): 324–343.

Littlewood, Ronald. "Psychiatric Diagnosis and Racial Bias: Empirical and Interpretative Approaches." *Social Science & Medicine* 34, no. 2 (January 1992): 141–149.

Litwack, Leon F. *North of Slavery: The Negro in the Free States, 1790–1860.* Chicago: University of Chicago Press, 1961.

———. *Trouble in Mind: Black Southerners in the Age of Jim Crow.* New York: Knopf, 1998.

Lockley, Timothy. *Welfare and Charity in the Antebellum South.* Gainesville: University of Florida Press, 2007.

Logan, Rayford W. *Howard University: The First Hundred Years 1867–1967.* New York: New York University Press, 1969.

Long, Gretchen. *Doctoring Freedom: The Politics of African American Medical Care in Slavery and Emancipation.* Chapel Hill: University of North Carolina Press, 2012.

Lorde, Audre. "The Uses of Anger: Women Responding to Racism." June 1981. *BlackPast,* August 12, 2012. http://www.blackpast.org/1981-audre-lorde-uses-anger-women-responding-racism.

Loring, Marti, and Brian Powell. "Gender, Race, and DSM-III: A Study of the Objectivity of Psychiatric Diagnostic Behavior." *Journal of Health and Social Behavior* 29, no. 1 (March 1988): 1–22.

Lowe, Richard. *Republicans and Reconstruction in Virginia, 1856–70.* Charlottesville: University of Virginia Press, 1991.

Mancini, Matthew J. *One Dies, Get Another: Convict Leasing in the American South, 1866–1928.* Columbia: University of South Carolina Press, 1996.

———. "Race, Economics, and the Abandonment of Convict Leasing." *Journal of Negro History* 63, no. 4 (1978): 339–352.

Marshall, Mary Louise. "Samuel A. Cartwright and States' Rights Medicine." *New Orleans Medical and Surgical Journal* 90 (August 1940): 74–78.

Martin, Michelle E. "Philosophical and Religious Influences on Social Welfare Policy in the United States: The Ongoing Effect of Reformed Theology and Social Darwinism on Attitudes Toward the Poor and Social Welfare Policy and Practice." *Journal of Social Work* 12, no. 1 (January 2012): 51–64.

Mason, Daniel, and Honor Hsin. "'A More Perfect Arrangement of Plants': The Botanical Model in Psychiatric Nosology, 1676 to the Present Day." *History of Psychiatry* 29, no. 2 (2018): 131–146.

McCandless, Peter. *Moonlight, Magnolias, and Madness: Insanity in South Carolina from the Colonial Period to the Progressive Era.* Chapel Hill: University of North Carolina Press, 1996.

———. *Slavery, Disease, and Suffering in the Southern Low Country.* Cambridge: Cambridge University Press, 2011.

McGovern, Constance. *Masters of Madness: Social Origins of the American Psychiatric Profession.* Burlington: University of Vermont Press, 1985.

McKee, Larry. "The Archaeological Study of Slavery and Plantation Life in Tennessee." *Tennessee Historical Quarterly* 59, no. 3 (Fall 2000): 188–203.

Meinke, Scott R. "Slavery, Partisanship, and Procedure in the U.S. House: The Gag Rule, 1836–1845." *Legislative Studies Quarterly* 32, no. 1 (2007): 33–58.

Melish, Joanne Pope. *Disowning Slavery: Gradual Emancipation and "Race" in New England, 1780–1860.* Ithaca, NY: Cornell University Press, 1998.

Mendes, Gabriel N. *Under the Strain of Color: Harlem's Lafargue Clinic and the Promise of an Antiracist Psychiatry.* Ithaca, NY: Cornell University Press, 2015.

Metzl, Jonathan. *The Protest Psychosis: How Schizophrenia Became a Black Disease.* Boston: Beacon, 2011.

Meyer, Manuella. *Reasoning Against Madness: Psychiatry and the State in Rio de Janeiro, 1830–1944.* Rochester, NY: University of Rochester Press, 2017.

Micale, Mark, and Roy Porter. *Discovering the History of Psychiatry.* Oxford: Oxford University Press, 1994.

Minardi, Margot. *Making Slavery History: Abolitionism and the Politics of Memory in Massachusetts.* Oxford: Oxford University Press, 2010.

———. "Making Slavery Visible (Again): The Nineteenth-Century Roots of a Revisionist Recovery in New England." In *Politics of Memory: Making Slavery Visible in the Public Space,* ed. Ana Lucia Araujo. London: Routledge, 2012.

Modak, Tamonud, Siddharth Sarkar, and Rajesh Sagar. "Dorothea Dix: A Proponent of Humane Treatment of Mentally Ill." *Journal of Mental Health and Human Behaviour* 21, no. 1 (January 2016): 69–71.

Morgan, Philip. *Slave Counterpoint: Black Culture in the Eighteenth-Century Chesapeake and Low Country.* Chapel Hill: University of North Carolina Press, 1998.

Morrison, Toni. *The Bluest Eye.* New York: Holt, Rinehart and Winston, 1970.

Moser Jones, Marian. "Creating a Science of Homelessness During the Reagan Era." *Milbank Quarterly* 93, no. 1 (March 2015): 139–178.

Mott, Frank Luther. *A History of American Magazines, 1850–1865.* Cambridge, MA: Harvard University Press, 1938.

Moulier Boutang, Yann. *De l'esclavage au salariat: économie historique du salariat bridé.* Paris: Presses Universitaires de France, 1998.

Murray, Pauli, ed. *States' Laws on Race and Color.* Athens: University of Georgia Press, 1997.

Myers, Bob. "Drapetomania: Rebellion, Defiance, and Free Black Insanity in the Antebellum United States." PhD diss., University of California Los Angeles, 2014.

Nobles, Melissa. *Shades of Citizenship: Race and the Census in Modern Politics.* Palo Alto, CA: Stanford University Press, 2000.

Novak, Daniel B. *The Wheel of Servitude: Black Forced Labor After Slavery.* Lexington: University Press of Kentucky, 1978.

O'Brien, M. J. *We Shall Not Be Moved: The Jackson Woolworth's Sit-In and the Movement It Inspired.* Jackson: University Press of Mississippi, 2013.

Ojalvo, Holly Epstein. "Beyond Yale: These Other University Buildings Have Ties to Slavery and White Supremacy." *USA Today,* February 13, 2017. https://eu.usatoday .com/story/college/2017/02/13/beyond-yale-these-other-university-buildings -have-ties-to-slavery-and-white-supremacy/37427471.

Olmstead, Alan L., and Paul W. Rhode. "Cotton, Slavery, and the New History of Capitalism." *Explorations in Economic History* 67 (January 2018): 1–17.

Oshinsky, David M. *Worse than Slavery: Parchman Farm and the Ordeal of Jim Crow Justice.* New York: The Free Press, 1996.

Osthaus, Carl. *Partisans of the Southern Press: Editorial Spokesmen of the Nineteenth Century.* Lexington: University Press of Kentucky, 2014.

Parry, Manon. "Dorothea Dix." *American Journal of Public Health* 96 (April 2006): 624–625.

Parsons, Elaine Frantz. *Ku-Klux: The Birth of the Klan During Reconstruction*. Chapel Hill: University of North Carolina Press, 2015.

Patterson, Orlando. *Slavery and Social Death: A Comparative Study*. Cambridge, MA: Harvard University Press, 1982.

Patterson, Thomas C. "An Archaeology of the History of Nineteenth-Century U.S. Anthropology: James McCune Smith, Radical Abolitionist and Anthropologist." *Journal of Anthropological Research* 69, no. 4 (2013): 459–484.

Pavkov, Thomas W., Dan A. Lewis, and John S. Lyons. "Psychiatric Diagnoses and Racial Bias: An Empirical Investigation." *Professional Psychology: Research and Practice* 20, no. 6 (December 1989): 364–368.

Peiretti-Courtis, Delphine. *Corps noirs et médecins blancs: La fabrique du préjugé racial, XIXe-XXe siècles*. Paris: La Découverte, 2021.

Porter, Theodore M. *The Rise of Statistical Thinking, 1820–1900*. Princeton, NJ: Princeton University Press, 1988.

Poskett, James. "Phrenology, Correspondence, and the Global Politics of Reform, 1815–1848." *Historical Journal* 60 (2017): 409–442.

Price, Gregory N., William Darity Jr., and Rhonda V. Sharpe. "Did North Carolina Economically Breed-Out Blacks During its Historical Eugenic Sterilization Campaign?" *American Review of Political Economy* 15, no. 1 (June 2020): 1–22.

Pride, Felicia. "Schizophrenia as Political Weapon." *The Root*, January 25, 2010. https://www.theroot.com/schizophrenia-as-political-weapon-1790878403.

Prieto, Leon C., and Simone T. A. Phipps. "Re-discovering Charles Clinton Spaulding's 'The Administration of Big Business': Insight into Early 20th Century African-American Management Thought." *Journal of Management History* 22, no. 1 (2016): 73–90.

Prochasson, Christophe, and Anne Rasmussen. "Du bon usage de la dispute. Introduction." *Mil neuf cent. Revue d'histoire intellectuelle* 25, no. 1 (February 2007): 5–12.

Rabier, Christelle. "The System of Professions, entre sociologie et histoire. Retour sur une recherche." In *Andrew Abbott et l'héritage de l'école de Chicago*, vol. 2, ed. Didier Demazière and Morgan Jouvenet, 320–339. Paris: Éditions de l'EHESS, 2016.

Rabinowitz, Howard. *Southern Black Leaders of the Reconstruction Era*. Urbana: University of Illinois Press, 1982.

Radzilowski, John. "Fecund Newcomers or Dying Ethnics? Demographic Approaches to the History of Polish and Italian Immigrants and Their Children in the United States, 1880 to 1980." *Journal of American Ethnic History* 27, no. 1 (Fall 2007): 60–74.

Randolph, Kirby Ann. "Central Lunatic Asylum for the Colored Insane: A History of African Americans with Mental Disabilities, 1844–1885." PhD diss., University of Pennsylvania, 2003.

Raz, Mical. *What's Wrong with the Poor? Psychiatry, Race, and the War on Poverty.* Chapel Hill: University of North Carolina Press, 2013.

Reed, Germaine A. "Race Legislation in Louisiana, 1864–1920." *Louisiana History: The Journal of the Louisiana Historical Association* 6, no. 4 (1965): 379–392.

Richardson, Joe M. "Florida Black Codes." *Florida Historical Quarterly* 47, no. 4 (April 1969): 365–379.

Riser, R. Volney. "Disfranchisement, the U.S. Constitution, and the Federal Courts: Alabama's 1901 Constitutional Convention Debates the Grandfather Clause." *American Journal of Legal History* 48, no. 3 (July 2006): 237–279.

Rodriguez, Junius P. "Always 'En Garde': The Effects of Slave Insurrection upon the Louisiana Mentality, 1811–1815." *Louisiana History: The Journal of the Louisiana Historical Association* 33, no. 4 (Autumn 1992): 399–416.

Rose, Anne C. *Psychology and Selfhood in the Segregated South.* Chapel Hill: University of North Carolina Press, 2009.

Rothman, David. *The Discovery of the Asylum: Social Order and Disorder in the New Republic.* Boston: Little, Brown, 1971.

Rothman, Joshua D. *Notorious in the Neighborhood: Sex and Families Across the Color Line in Virginia, 1787–1861.* Chapel Hill: University of North Carolina Press, 2003.

Ruiz, Pedro, and Annelle Primm, eds. *Disparities in Psychiatric Care: Clinical and Cross-Cultural Perspectives.* Baltimore: Lippincott Williams & Wilkins, 2010.

Samson, Colin. "Inequality, the New Right and Mental Health Care Delivery in the United States in the Reagan Era." *Critical Social Policy* 10, no. 29 (October 1990): 40–57.

Satz, Ronald. *Tennessee's Indian Peoples: From White Contact to Removal, 1540–1840.* Knoxville: University of Tennessee Press, 1979.

Savitt, Todd. *Medicine and Slavery: The Diseases and Health Care of Blacks in Antebellum Virginia.* Champaign: University of Illinois Press, 1978.

———. "The Use of Blacks for Medical Experimentation and Demonstration in the Old South." *Journal of Southern History* 48, no. 3 (1982): 331–348.

Schiebinger, Londa. "The Anatomy of Difference: Race and Sex in Eighteenth-Century Science." *Eighteenth-Century Studies* 23, no. 4 (Summer 1990): 387–405.

———. *Secret Cures of Slaves: People, Plants, and Medicine in the Eighteenth-Century Atlantic World.* Palo Alto, CA: Stanford University Press, 2017.

Schoen, Joanna. "Between Choice and Coercion: Women and the Politics of Sterilization in North Carolina, 1929–1975." *Journal of Women's History* 13, no. 1 (Spring 2001): 132–156.

Schor, Paul. *Counting Americans: How the U.S. Census Classified the Nation,* trans. Lys Ann Weiss. New York: Oxford University Press, 2017.

———. "The Disappearance of the 'Mulatto' as the End of Inquiry into the Composition of the Black Population of the United States," in *Counting Americans: How the U.S. Census Classified the Nation,* trans. Lys Ann Weiss, 158–168 (New York: Oxford University Press, 2017).

Scull, Andrew. "From Madness to Mental Illness: Medical Men as Moral Entrepreneurs." *European Journal of Sociology* 16, no. 2 (1975): 218–251.

Segrest, Mab. *Administrations of Lunacy: Racism and the Haunting of American Psychiatry at the Milledgeville Asylum.* New York: The New Press, 2020.

Seraile, William. "The Brief Diplomatic Career of Henry Highland Garnet." *Phylon* 46, no. 1 (1985): 71–81.

Shapiro, Herbert. *White Violence and Black Response: From Reconstruction to Montgomery.* Amherst: University of Massachusetts Press, 1988.

Sheehan-Dean, Aaron, ed. *A Companion to the U.S. Civil War.* New York: John Wiley & Sons, 2014.

Sheppard, Elizabeth. "Problème public." In *Dictionnaire des politiques publiques. 3ᵉ édition actualisée et augmentée,* ed. Laurie Boussaquet, Sophie Jacquot, and Pauline Ravinet, 530–538. Paris: Presses de Sciences Po, 2010.

Shklar, Judith N. *American Citizenship: The Quest for Inclusion.* Cambridge, MA: Harvard University Press, 1991.

Siegel, Frederick H. *The Roots of Southern Distinctiveness: Tobacco and Society in Danville, Virginia, 1780–1865.* Chapel Hill: University of North Carolina Press, 1987.

Smith, Sean Morey, and Christopher D. E. Willoughby, eds. *Medicine and Healing in the Age of Slavery.* Baton Rouge: Louisiana State University Press, 2021.

Sommerville, Diane Miller. *Rape and Race in the Nineteenth-Century South.* Chapel Hill: University of North Carolina Press, 2004.

Stanton, William. *The Leopard's Spots: Scientific Attitudes Toward Race in America, 1815–59.* Chicago: University of Chicago Press, 1960.

Stefani, Anne. *Unlikely Dissenters: White Southern Women in the Fight for Racial Justice, 1920–1970.* Gainesville: University Press of Florida, 2015.

Stowe, Steven M. *Doctoring the South: Southern Physicians and Everyday Medicine in the Mid-Nineteenth Century.* Chapel Hill, University of North Carolina Press, 2004.

Summers, Martin. "Diagnosing the Ailments of Black Citizenship: The African American Medical Profession and the Politics of Mental Illness, 1895–1940." In *Precarious Prescriptions: Contested Histories of Race and Health in North America,* ed. Laurie Green, John McKiernan-Gonzalez, and Martin Summers, 91–114. Minneapolis: University of Minnesota Press, 2014.

————. *Madness in the City of Magnificent Intentions: A History of Race and Mental Illness in the Nation's Capital.* New York: Oxford University Press, 2019.

————. "Suitable Care of the African When Afflicted With Insanity: Race, Madness, and Social Order in Comparative Perspective." *Bulletin of the History of Medicine* 84, no. 1 (Spring 2010): 58–91.

Summerville, James. *Educating Black Doctors: A History of Meharry Medical College.* Tuscaloosa: University of Alabama Press, 2002.

Szasz, Thomas. *The Myth of Mental Illness.* New York: Hoeber-Harper, 1961.

Taylor, A. A. "Historians of the Reconstruction." *Journal of Negro History* 23 (January 1938): 16–34.

Thomas, Alexander, and Samuel Sillen. *Racism and Psychiatry.* New York: Brunner/Mazel, 1972.

Thomas, Karen Kruse. *Deluxe Jim Crow: Civil Rights and American Health Policy, 1935–1954.* Athens: University of Georgia Press, 2011.

Thompson, E. P. "The Moral Economy of the English Crowd in the Eighteenth Century." *Past & Present* 50 (February 1971): 76–136.

Tolnay, Stewart E., and E. M. Beck. *A Festival of Violence: An Analysis of Southern Lynchings, 1882–1930.* Urbana: University of Illinois Press, 1992.

Tregle, Joseph G., Jr. "Early New Orleans Society: A Reappraisal." *Journal of Southern History* 18 (February 1952): 20–36.

Turner Censer, Jane. *The Reconstruction of White Southern Womanhood, 1865–1895.* Baton Rouge: Louisiana State University Press, 2003.

Vesely-Flad, Rima L. *Racial Purity and Dangerous Bodies: Moral Pollution, Black Lives, and the Struggle for Justice.* Minneapolis: Fortress Press, 2017.

Vidal, Cécile. *Louisiana: Crossroads of the Atlantic World.* Philadelphia: University of Pennsylvania Press, 2014.

Vincent, Charles. *Black Legislators in Louisiana During Reconstruction.* Baton Rouge: Louisiana State University Press, 1976.

Wacquant, Loïc. "Deadly Symbiosis: When Ghetto and Prison Meet and Mesh." *Punishment & Society* 3, no. 1 (2001): 95–133.

Wagner, David. *The Poorhouse: America's Forgotten Institution.* New York: Rowman and Littlefield, 2005.

Wailoo, Keith. *Dying in the City of the Blues: Sickle Cell Anemia and the Politics of Race and Health.* Chapel Hill: University of North Carolina Press, 2014.

Waller, Altina L. "Community, Class and Race in the Memphis Riot of 1866." *Journal of Social History* 18, no. 2 (Winter 1984): 233–246.

Ward, Thomas J. *Black Physicians in the Jim Crow South.* Fayetteville: University of Arkansas Press, 2003.

Washington, Harriet A. *Medical Apartheid: The Dark History of Medical Experimentation on Black Americans from Colonial Times to the Present*. New York: Knopf Doubleday, 2008.

Weiner, Dora B. "Betrayal! The 1806 English Translation of Pinel's traité médico-philosophique sur l'aliénation mentale ou la manie." *Gesnerus* 57 (2000): 42–50.

Weiner, Marli F., and Mazie Hough. *Sex, Sickness, and Slavery Illness in the Antebellum South*. Champaign: University of Illinois Press, 2012.

Whaley, Arthur L. "Ethnicity/Race, Paranoia, and Psychiatric Diagnoses: Clinician Bias Versus Sociocultural Differences." *Journal of Psychopathology and Behavioral Assessment* 19, no. 1 (March 1997): 1–20.

Wiley, Bell I. "Southern Reaction to Federal Invasion." *Journal of Southern History* 16, no. 4 (November 1950): 491–510.

Williams, Eric. *Capitalism and Slavery*. Chapel Hill: University of North Carolina Press, 1994.

Willoughby, Christopher. "Running Away from Drapetomania: Samuel Cartwright, Medicine, and Race in the Antebellum South." *Journal of Southern History* 84, no. 3 (August 2018): 579–614.

Wish, Harvey. "The Slave Insurrection Panic of 1856." *Journal of Southern History* 5, no. 2 (May 1939): 206–227.

Wood, Amy Louise. "Lynching Photography and the Visual Reproduction of White Supremacy." *American Nineteenth Century History* 6, no. 3 (2005): 373–399.

Woodard, Vincent. *The Delectable Negro: Human Consumption and Homoeroticism Within U.S. Slave Culture*. New York: New York University Press, 2014.

Woodward, C. Vann. *The Origins of the New South*. Baton Rouge: Louisiana State University Press, 1951.

Young, Harvey. "The Black Body as Souvenir in American Lynching." *Theatre Journal* 57, no. 4 (December 2005): 639–657.

Index

Adler, Alfred, 16, 136, 153–156. *See also* European psychoanalysts

African American women: and childbirth, 36, 102, 106; as performing gender-specific tasks, 36, 121–124, 127, 132; as pictured in photographs, 9, 87, 88; protesting enslavement, 22; seen as affected by specific diseases, 24, 100, 105–106; and sexual violence, 140, 143–145, 191n32; and sleeping arrangements in hospitals, 86–87; as stereotyped, 3, 15, 140, 152, 165n7; and sterilization, 94

Alabama, 1, 24, 32, 46, 82, 91, 109, 116, 142, 144

alienation: as a form of repression, 11; mental, 31, 44, 96, 109, 114, 130, 143

American Anti-Slavery Society, 56, 58

American Journal of Insanity: founding of, 8, 12; and publications on race, 61, 108, 154

Americanization, 106, 134–135

Andrews, Judson B., 15, 108–109

Annales médico-psychologiques, 53

annual reports: and budgets, 88–90, 93; photographs in, 124; and segregation, 80, 127–130

anti-abolitionism, 27–28, 41, 103, 160, 170n24

anti-immigrant rhetoric: and labor, 102–103; and madness, 106–108; and southern political culture, 117

Arkansas, 34, 81, 92, 144

Baldwin, James, 1–3, 159

Baldwin, Robert F., 67–68, 82

Barkdull, James D., 58, 64–65

benevolent associations, 76

Bevis, William, 138, 143, 148

black agency: and resistance to enslavement, 32, 34, 65, 103, 125, 160; and resistance to systemic violence, 2, 7, 11, 14–15, 157, 178n22; and strategies of resistance against forced labor, 15, 99, 128, 129, 130, 132

black education: lack of funding for, 82–84; and patients, 100, 155; schools in black communities, 69, 73, 79; and segregation, 91; and theories on technical training, 118–119, 131

Black Lives Matter, 162

black men and women: as dangerous, 3, 13, 36, 49, 65, 103, 117, 141; as indocile, 7, 15, 83, 98, 103, 123, 128; as infantile, 36, 110, 135, 147–152, 157; as naive, 152

black suffrage: and black voters, 91, 104, 54n181; and violence, 69, 91

Bleeding Kansas, 61

Brown, H. Rap, 3

Caldwell, Charles: and monogenism, 13n169; and phrenology, 52

Calhoun, John C.: and the census, 51; opposition to free Blacks in New York, 55–59; and the supposed inferiority of certain races, 52

capitalism, 122, 172n48, 187n69

Carmichael, Stokely, 3

Cartwright, Samuel: advocate for the rise of the medical profession in the South, 25–29, 43–44, 105; and the Fugitive Slave Act of 1850, 20; and manual labor, 34–35;

CPSIA information can be obtained
at www.ICGtesting.com
Printed in the USA
LVHW101602010223
738413LV00003B/63